Assessing
Veterinary Nurses
in Practice

For Elsevier:

Commissioning Editor: Mary Seager
Development Editor: Rita Demetriou-Swanwick
Project Manager: Caroline Horton
Designer: Andy Chapman

Assessing Veterinary Nurses in Practice

Jill Diana Warner CertEd VN D32 33 34 35

VNAC Co-ordinator and Internal Verifier
Norton Radstock College, Bath, UK

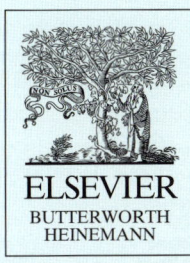

ELSEVIER
BUTTERWORTH
HEINEMANN

Edinburgh   London   New York   Oxford   Philadelphia   St Louis   Sydney   Toronto   2005

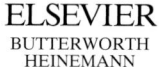

ELSEVIER
BUTTERWORTH
HEINEMANN

First published 2005
ISBN 0 7506 8840 8

British Library Cataloguing in Publication Data
A catalogue record for this book is available from the British Library

Library of Congress Cataloging in Publication Data
A catalog record for this book is available from the Library of Congress

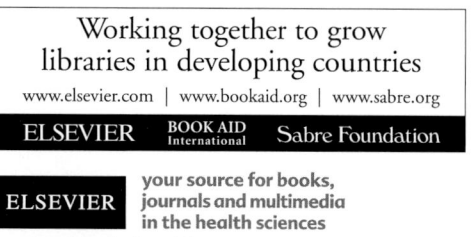

Working together to grow
libraries in developing countries

www.elsevier.com | www.bookaid.org | www.sabre.org

ELSEVIER   BOOK AID International   Sabre Foundation

ELSEVIER your source for books,
journals and multimedia
in the health sciences
www.elsevierhealth.com

The
Publisher's
policy is to use
**paper manufactured
from sustainable forests**

Printed in China

Contents

CHAPTER 5   **External Organizations**   **141**

CHAPTER 6   **Developments in the Veterinary Nursing Profession**   **145**

CD Contents

Allocation plan
Appeals procedure
Assessment plan – Word and Excel
Assessor paperwork checklist
Assessor standardization meeting questionnaire
Curriculum vitae
Feedback record – Word and Excel
Internal verification communication record
Internal verification approval and monitoring visit checklist
Internal verification assessor support form
Internal verification report form – Word and Excel
Internal verification of assessment sampling grid
Training practice tracking matrix

Acknowledgements

Thanks to:

Kelly Russell EVN of the Bell Equine Veterinary Clinic, Kent for her advice regarding the equine case logs.

Cover photography courtesy of Jill Warner and Donna Morse, with grateful acknowledgement to Pippa Dawkins, Tina Tucker, Natalya Knowles and Trevor Warner.

Preface

It would not be unreasonable to assume that if you are reading this you are involved in assessing student veterinary nurses or verifying the assessment process itself. How this involvement came about varies from those with an inherent passion for veterinary nurse training to those who have been coerced into the role because no one else either wants it or is available to undertake it!

Whichever the case, my hope is that you will find this book useful as a guide. Even if you decide not to read it from cover to cover, you may dip into it and glean information, guidance and support from the pages herein. Although NVQ students are referred to as 'candidates', I will use the term 'student' throughout this book as within our profession we have student veterinary nurses. Regardless of whether your students are training to become small animal veterinary nurses or equine nurses, the principles behind being an assessor are exactly the same. I have included example small animal and equine case logs. All references to the portfolio and occupational standards are current at the time of writing. However, the award is to be re-accredited in 2006 and some of the nomenclature may well change.

Formal assessment of students within the veterinary practice is vitally important for both the student and the practice alike. First, it enables a student's level of competence to be officially identified, even if this means confirming that in fact the person is not yet competent. Second, regardless of the outcome of the assessment, both the assessor and the student immediately know what they are capable of doing in terms of the practical ability to perform nursing tasks. Third, it identifies the depth of the student's underpinning knowledge. From students' point of view, this protects them from being expected to undertake tasks that they are not yet competent to perform and also provides the necessary confirmation the practice needs before allowing students to undertake more responsibility.

Jill Warner 2005

The History and Evolution of Veterinary Nurse Training

1961: the Registered Animal Nursing Auxiliary (RANA) was born

Following the formation of the British Small Animal Veterinary Association (BSAVA) in 1957, this new association rapidly recognized the importance of nursing assistance in small animal practices. The Royal College of Veterinary Surgeons (RCVS) was approached by the association to instigate a training scheme in 1961. In that year, recognition was given for the first time for those working in veterinary practice by crediting them for their experience and expertise of nursing skills. March 1965 saw the formation of the British Veterinary Nursing Association (BVNA) with 30 RANAs and Animal Nursing Auxiliary (ANA) trainees as members. Consistency of training was endeavoured through traditional methods of external assessment (i.e. written and practical examinations). However, this method had its limitations because of the different interpretation of standards within individual practices.

1984: the title 'veterinary nurse' came into being

A change in legislation in 1979 in the Nurses, Midwives and Health Visitors Act removed the protection of the title of 'nurse' for use solely for members of the General Nursing Council. As a result the title veterinary nurse (VN) was permitted to be used, although this was not enacted until 1984. Where training was concerned, consistency continued via the use of traditional methods of external assessment, but there remained the difficulty of individual interpretation of standards in practices.

In addition, in the 1980s, media attention resulted in an increased expectation of VNs. The popular 'Vet's in Practice' and 'RSPCA' series on television, together with the *Animal Ark* books written by Lucy Daniels, demonstrated and highlighted the role of the VN in practice.

1999 Scottish/National Vocational Qualifications

January 1999 saw the introduction of the Veterinary Nursing Scottish and National Vocational Qualification (S/NVQ). Consistency was again ensured by maintaining traditional methods of external assessment; with the introduction of formal workplace assessment; this should mean improved working practice throughout the profession.

As with the implementation of any new S/NVQ, initially there were insufficient numbers of qualified or experienced assessors as well as a lack of internal verifiers (IVs) progressing within the system. The problem of individual practices having differing interpretations of working standards still posed a problem for the Royal College of Veterinary Surgeons (RCVS) as the awarding body. This, coupled with a lack of appropriate levels of support provided for the assessors owing to the large number of Approved Training and Assessment Centres (ATACs) throughout the country, meant something had to be done.

In response to this, in 2001, the RCVS introduced the Veterinary Nursing Approved Centre (VNAC) and Training and Assessment Practice (TP) in order to develop quality assurance and standardization and to maintain support for assessors and internal verifiers with the NVQ structure. The VNAC employs internal verifiers who are responsible for approving, monitoring and supporting the TPs, who employ assessors to assess students in the workplace. The TPs have replaced the old ATACs. In doing so, the RCVS followed the tier system as usually found within S/NVQ work-based assessment models (see Box 1.1).

The awarding body employs external verifiers (EVs) who liaise directly with the IVs within the VNACs. The IVs in turn have direct regular contact with the assessors working in the TPs who have joined and become affiliated with their VNAC, thus ensuring that any information and guidance from the awarding body is disseminated from EV to IV, from the IV to assessors and from the assessors to their students.

In 2002 SVQs were phased out because of the small number of students in Scotland accessing these awards. The RCVS could not justify the associated expense and administration of accreditation with a second regulatory authority; therefore the remainder of this book will refer only to NVQs.

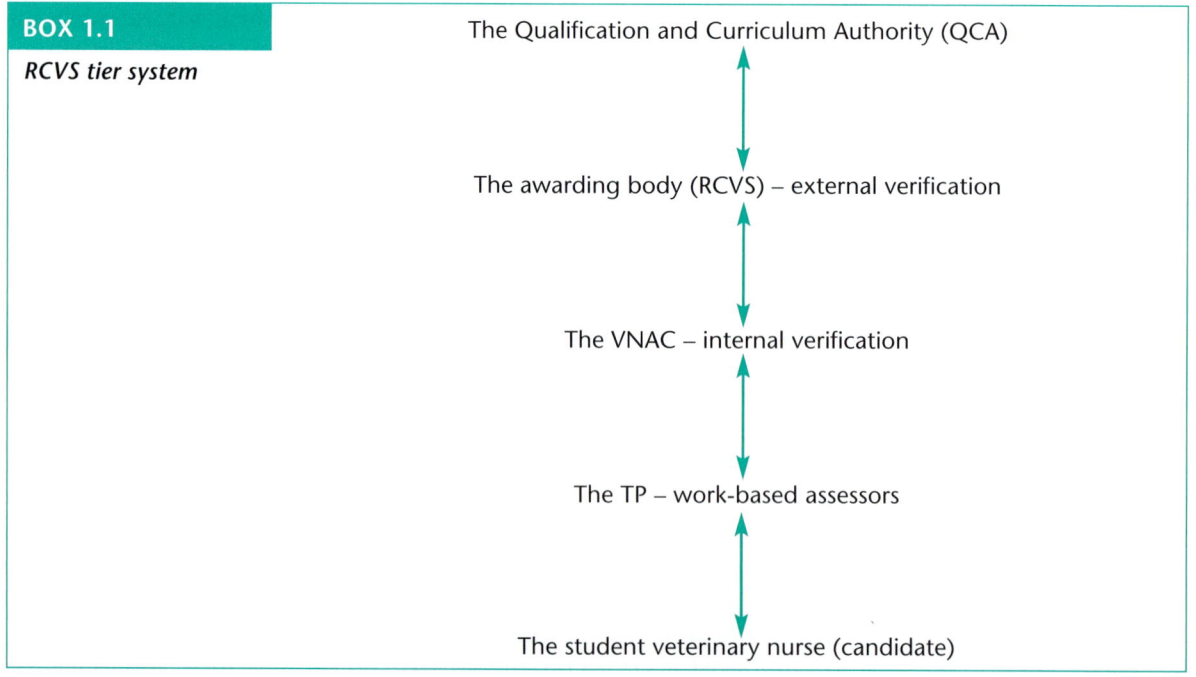

BOX 1.1

RCVS tier system

The Qualification and Curriculum Authority (QCA)

The awarding body (RCVS) – external verification

The VNAC – internal verification

The TP – work-based assessors

The student veterinary nurse (candidate)

The veterinary nursing NVQ system ensures the following:

- *Consistency*: this is achieved by maintaining the traditional methods of external assessment, which involve multiple choice question examinations at both level 2 and level 3 together with practical exams at level 3. Effective monitoring of training and course provision is ensured through internal and external verification, which is provided by the VNAC and RCVS, respectively.

- *Improved working practices*: although student nurses were always observed working in their training practice, workplace assessment became formalized with the implementation of the veterinary nursing NVQ. It is monitored by IVs who visit assessors and students in their training practices to offer support and guidance and to verify the assessment process. This ensures that all students are being assessed to the same standards and are provided with equal opportunity for assessment. Previously students had to be observed only once carrying out a series of set tasks; often they were literally observed on one occasion for each task, which did not confirm they had received sufficient training or demonstrate their underpinning knowledge or ongoing competence at performing a task.

Consistency of standards within TPs is being reviewed and will be improved further with the implementation of the RCVS Practice Standards Scheme in January 2005. This is a voluntary scheme that replaces the BSAVA approved practices and British Veterinary Hospital Association (BVHA)/RCVS Veterinary Hospitals with a three-tier system where veterinary practices are inspected and awarded the relevant tier for approval. Following initial approval, these practices will be inspected every 4 years by a team of veterinary surgeon inspectorates. Spot checks are also planned and those practices at tier 2, which are actively training nurses, will continue to be monitored and supported by internal verifiers from their VNAC. The emphasis on IV visits will then purely relate to training; however, liaison between the IV and RCVS will be expected where necessary. The general public will be made aware of the relevance of each tier through advertising campaigns. A practice awarded tier 1 will comply with core standards that mainly relate to legal and health and safety requirements. Tier 2 covers both small animal and farm and equine practices, and includes the standards already required by TPs for veterinary nurse training. Tier 3 practices may be either small animal or equine and will comply with veterinary hospital standards. Each practice will display a practice standards certificate enabling clients to know which tier they have been awarded. The system is designed to increase general client awareness and confidence in veterinary practice.

Assessor Training

THE ASSESSMENT STRATEGY

The Assessment Strategy document was produced by Lantra, the Sector Skills Council responsible for veterinary nursing in November 2001, following consultation with the industry including representatives from the RCVS, BVNA, BSAVA, general practices and training providers. A copy of this document can be obtained via the RCVS website (www.rcvs.org.uk) or Lantra (www.lantra.co.uk). The document spells out the requirements for being an assessor, internal verifier and external verifier for veterinary nursing and provides information regarding workplace assessment and the use of simulation.

The Assessment Strategy stipulates that an assessor must be either a qualified veterinary surgeon or a listed veterinary nurse and be occupationally competent, that is, capable of carrying out the role as an assessor in accordance with the new Employment National Training Organization (ENTO) unit A1 assessor award. Those who have already achieved the TDLB D32 and D33 assessor awards will not be required to requalify but will be equivalent to A1 assessors and be expected to assess to the standards set out in the A1 award.

The Assessment Strategy also stipulates that all veterinary surgeons and nurses should have a minimum of 1 year's postqualification experience prior to undertaking assessor training. This may be frustrating to the enthusiastic and aspiring assessor; however this decision was made for good reasons. The majority of veterinary nurse training is undertaken over a 2- or 2½-year timescale, by students generally remaining in one training practice. The breadth and depth of experience can therefore in itself be quite limiting and newly qualified veterinary nurses or veterinary surgeons need to be able to draw on their own clinical experience to support students and assess their competence. Students also need the support and guidance from an assessor who has been actively engaged in continuing professional development (CPD) and who has the maturity and respect to be able to make decisions about the competency of a student, especially when the student has not met the national

---

An assessor must:

- be either a veterinary surgeon or a listed veterinary nurse
- be qualified for at least a year before undertaking assessor training
- either hold or be working towards the D32 and 33 or A1 assessor awards
- undertake CPD.

standard. If all is going well, it may appear easy to assess, but it can be difficult when students really believe they have met the national standard and you know they have not. Examples of assessment scenarios and giving feedback are included later in this chapter under 'Giving feedback'.

DEVELOPING AND SUPPORTING THE ASSESSOR THROUGH TRAINING AND BEYOND

In exactly the same way as student veterinary nurses have to demonstrate that they can meet the nursing Occupational Standards (i.e. be assessed as competent), trainee assessors have to compile evidence to demonstrate they have met the standards for being an assessor. As such, many assessors in TPs have already achieved the Training and Development Lead Body's (TDLB) D32 and D33 assessor awards. D32 'Assess candidate performance' involved observing student veterinary nurses' practical skills and assessing their performance. D33 'Assess candidate using differing sources of evidence' involved assessing other types of evidence produced by students – such as the case logs within their portfolios and answers to oral and written questions devised by assessors as a means to determine their students' level of underpinning knowledge. Ideally, D32/33 trainee assessors should have assessed two or three different students to provide evidence of how they planned, assessed and provided feedback to inexperienced students, students with special assessment requirements and experienced students. However, in small practices where there was only one student nurse, students were assessed at different stages of their training as they would have had different assessment needs as they progressed through the award.

These two D units have been superseded by the new ENTO unit A1 assessor award, which qualifies the assessor to 'Assess students using a range of methods', that is, observation, written evidence, etc.

Training for the A1 award

(Additional information can be found at www.empnto.co.uk.)

A trainee A1 assessor must provide evidence of assessing a minimum of two students. Those within small practices with access to only one student veterinary nurse will need to speak to their assessor tutor or VNAC to gain advice. The options suggested by the RCVS include:

- assessing a VN student at a branch TP of the same practice
- the VNAC arranging access to a VN student at another affiliated TP
- assessing an animal care student at a local college using its specific occupational standards.

The students being assessed must be enrolled students so that any evidence collected by the trainee assessor relating to the assessment can theoretically be used by students as evidence towards their own qualification.

The A1 unit is written in easier language than D32/33 and is broken down into four elements:

A1.1 Develop plans for assessing competence with candidates

A1.2 Judge evidence against criteria to make assessment decisions

A1.3 Provide feedback and support to candidates on assessment decisions

A1.4 Contribute to the internal quality assurance process.

Each element is broken down and stipulates exactly what is required by the assessor. The individual performance criteria within each of the four elements have been reworded to help you interpret their meaning. It is recommended that you read these together with the original copy supplied by your tutor:

A1.1

This involves assessors planning an assessment in advance and deciding what unit(s) and element(s) from the VN Occupational Standards they are going to assess their students on.

a. Assessors should plan and discuss an assessment with the student in advance of the day on which it will take place.

b. Assessors should ensure students are aware of the actual assessment process, the level of support they should expect to receive from their assessor and the fact that they have the right to appeal against any assessment decision if they don't agree with it. Students must also be aware of their TP's appeals policy.

c. All assessment methods must be:
   fair – be impartial when assessing and ensure you assess all of your students, not just the 'easy' or enthusiastic ones
   safe – ensure health and safety is maintained at all times in relation to both humans and animals
   valid – ensure the assessment is relevant to the VN Occupational Standards and only assess students at their appropriate level (e.g. level 2 or level 3)
   reliable – ensure the evidence reflects a level of performance consistently demonstrated by students in their work.

d. Evidence should be naturally occurring during the normal working day; therefore assessments should be planned when both the assessor and student are at work and ideally on the same shift.

e. To assess different types of evidence, assessors should plan to observe the student carrying out a practical task, ask oral questions and set written questions, etc.

f. Assessors should take into account what students have just learnt at college, and not assess them on topics they have not yet covered; if they have already achieved level 2 then assess them only at level 3.

g. Assessors should talk to the students about their needs and identify any specific assessment requirements they may have. In one TP, a student had recently broken her foot and therefore she needed to be able to sit down while being assessed. Other special requirements may include: dyslexia, colour blindness, hearing impairment, anxiety/nervousness, additional staff present such as an IV or EV. More details on planning for special arrangements are provided in the next chapter.

h. While working alongside a student, other qualified vets and nurses who do not hold an assessor award can act as a witness or evidence gatherer and make a statement on how the student performed. It is essential to let a potential evidence gatherer know what is expected of them before they actually observe a student. An assessor should show them the standards beforehand and also discuss the case with them afterwards to ascertain how the student performed.

i. Both client and candidate confidentiality must be maintained at all times. Client personal details should be deleted from all documentation and copies of any paperwork relating to a student's assessment must be kept locked away, with only those involved having access to them.

j. Assessors should be open with students and let them know that if they are not happy with any aspect of the assessment process, they can discuss this. Having a good relationship with the student(s) will help here! Every TP must have an appeals policy.

k. All those involved in an assessment must agree in advance when it is going to take place. This may involve additional people such as a client or other colleagues.

l. Regardless of the outcome of an assessment, it is essential to review the student's progress. For example, if the assessment went well, it may be necessary to check in a few months' time that the student is still competent or is competent to carry out the same task but with a different species. If the student was not competent, a review date should be set for reassessment.

m. Assessors should identify further training requirements to meet the student's needs, taking into account which occupational standards they have already met and those that remain outstanding.

A1.2

This involves assessors making a judgement or decision on the evidence produced by their students against the Occupational Standards – that is, whether or not they have met the national standard.

Assessors must demonstrate the following:

a. Whatever method of assessment is agreed on with the student must be adhered to. For example, if you agree on a practical assessment only, do not suddenly ask the student to answer written questions.

b. Assessors should identify the students' current level of competence both practically and theoretically and then use this as a baseline to decide what to assess them on. Similarly, if students were assessed several months ago, it is reasonable to reassess them to ensure they are still competent at an earlier task, particularly if they have exams in the near future.

c. All evidence must be authentic, that is, produced by the student. Observing a student's practical performance will provide such evidence. Any written evidence should be signed by students to confirm it as their own. However, if assessors are unsure as to the authenticity of any evidence, this should be discussed with students and if necessary questions asked around the topic to determine the level of their knowledge.

d. Assessment decisions must be based on the following criteria:
   safe – assessors should ensure the student maintains health and safety at all times in relation to both humans and animals
   fair – assessors should ensure they assess the student against the agreed criteria and Occupational Standards
   valid – assessors should ensure the assessment is relevant to the VN Occupational Standards and assess students only at their appropriate level (e.g. level 2 or level 3)
   reliable – ensure the evidence is the students' own work and reflects a level of performance consistently demonstrated in their work.

e. Assessors should discuss the student's performance with any witnesses or evidence gatherers who took part in the assessment.

f. If, when discussing the assessment with the student any special arrangements were agreed, assessors should write these down as part of the plan itself and then make sure they are carried out.

g. Assessors should remember to look at all the evidence; it may be that the student was not practically competent but answered all the questions well thus demonstrating excellent underpinning knowledge. In this case only the practical task should be reassessed.

h. If any of the evidence students produce is not to an expected standard (i.e. they are believed to be very competent at performing a particular task, but during the assessment are unable to do so), assessors should discuss this with them. This enables them to take ownership and identify any errors themselves. If they think it went well but they clearly have not met the national standard, this must be explained to them, remembering to give positive feedback as well as constructive advice as to ways of achieving the national standards next time. This may involve the assessor identifying specific further training requirements for the student, for example going on a CPD course or a revision course.

i. Assessors should keep records of all assessment decisions and any feedback given to students. The internal verifier will advise on which documentation to complete in line with the requirements of the awarding body.

j. If a disagreement arises between an assessor and a student regarding an assessment decision, this must be discussed with the relevant people. All students and assessors must be aware of the appeals policy within their TP. (An example is provided at the end of this section.)

A1.3

This involves the assessor providing feedback and support to the student regarding assessment decisions.

The actual performance criteria state:

a. Feedback should always be given as soon after the assessment as possible. We often remember things with rose-coloured spectacles and, unless we discuss things at the time, it is easy to forget exactly what happened during a practical assessment. Feedback should not be given in front of other people, unless relevant (i.e. internal or external verifiers); therefore, it may be more appropriate to move to a different place for the discussion.

b. Feedback must always be constructive and be aimed at the student's level of confidence. As mentioned earlier, if assessors ask the students how they feel the assessment went before giving any feedback, regardless of whether they have met the national standards or not, this encourages them to reflect on their own practice/knowledge and, where necessary, identify any errors they may have made or things they think they should have done differently. As a relationship develops with the students and they become more experienced with the assessment process and their nursing skills and knowledge develop, assessors and students should both find the giving and receiving of feedback easier.

c. Following initial feedback, assessors should give students further positive comments on their performance or written evidence, or both. They should follow this by identifying any aspects of the assessment that have not met the national standards.

d. It is important to help students identify ways in which they can achieve the national standard by discussing the evidence needed to do so. It may be necessary for them to practise the task more to gain sufficient competence or to undertake further reading around a subject to gain sufficient underpinning knowledge.

e. If a student needs clarification or further explanation about the initial feedback, assessors should discuss this with them in more detail.

f. Part of the feedback process is to agree a review date following any assessment. This will depend on the outcome of the assessment itself. If the national standards were met, the date for reviewing students' practical competence and underpinning knowledge may be in several months' time or sooner if, say, evidence of them nursing another species is required. If the student was not considered competent, a date for a further assessment must be agreed giving the student sufficient time to gain the necessary skills and knowledge needed.

g. All staff involved in the assessment process must be aware of the appeals policy within the practice and this must be followed in the event of a student having a complaint or appealing against an assessment decision.

A1.4

This involves the assessor providing evidence for the internal verifier to monitor quality assurance.

a. It is essential to keep written evidence of all assessment records, tutorial records, etc. to meet with the awarding body requirements. These provide evidence that assessors are actually doing their job!

b. Attending standardization sessions or workshops and discussing the assessment process with others is a very beneficial way for assessors to ensure they are both up to date and making correct assessment decisions.

c. All documented evidence relating to assessments must be completed as near to the date of the assessment as possible and be duly signed and dated by both student and assessor to authenticate them.

d. Quality assurance ensures that all students are assessed fairly and that assessment decisions in the workplace meet the national standard. The internal verifier will inform assessors of the awarding body requirements for ensuring compliance with the quality assurance process. This will also involve keeping records, attending meetings, etc.

Box 2.1 is an example of an appeals policy that may be used; alternatively, the internal verifier from the VNAC will be able to provide one.

In addition to demonstrating a practical ability to assess students and keep documented evidence of the assessments, assessors will have to provide evidence of their underpinning knowledge of 'the nature and role of assessments of competence', 'principles and concepts' and 'external factors influencing the assessment of national standards'. The knowledge

BOX 2.1 *Appeals procedure*	Should a student veterinary nurse disagree with the assessment decision made by one of the assessors within the practice, the student may appeal against such a decision by following the procedures below:

1. The student should discuss the assessment results with the assessor within 5 days of the assessment taking place, in the hope that a satisfactory conclusion can be met.

2. If either the student or the assessor feels unable to reach a satisfactory conclusion within 7 days, advice should be sought from the IV.

3. The IV will investigate the appeal, make a decision and report to the mentor within 7 days. However, if the student does not agree with this decision, then a full appeal can be instigated by following the procedures below:
   a. The student should notify the mentor about the wish to appeal within 48 hours of receiving the IV's report.
   b. The mentor should then liaise with the IV and the case is handed to the practice principal.
   c. The practice principal should convene an appeals panel to judge the appeal.
   d. The appeals panel will meet and consider the appeal. The practice principal should inform the student, assessor and IV of the panel's decision in writing within 7 days.

The EV should be noted at all stages described above.

requirements will be provided by the A1 assessor tutor together with a list of questions. Answering these questions correctly will demonstrate your underpinning knowledge and provide the necessary evidence accordingly.

Before going on to look at how to plan and write an assessment, we will look at how to interpret and use the Occupational Standards in relation to the assessment process and monitoring of students' progress.

THE OCCUPATIONAL STANDARDS

These are the most important documents in the assessment process as they stipulate exactly what a student VN must be able to demonstrate practically together with the underpinning knowledge they need to have to be competent and achieve both level 2 and level 3 of the veterinary nursing NVQ. The original version of the VN Occupational Standards was written in what can only be described as typical NVQ 'speak' giving rise to confused trainee assessors who initially spent hours trying to interpret them. Fortunately these were rewritten following the same consultation process as the Assessment Strategy and the current version was approved by Lantra in January 2002. We now have a more 'user friendly' and easier to interpret set of standards that sets out for students, assessors and verifiers exactly what the students are expected to do in terms of performance, the depth of knowledge and understanding they must demonstrate and the scope or breadth of the syllabus that they are expected to cover. These are available on disc or as a hard copy and can be obtained from the Lantra website or from the RCVS.

All newly enrolled student veterinary nurses (SVNs) are automatically provided with the 3rd edition portfolio and current Occupational Standards. Any SVN who was certificated for level 2 after 1 August 2002 must also be using edition 3 of the portfolio along with the latest Occupational Standards.

Using the Occupational Standards

As the name suggests, these identify what assessors actually assess their students against, in order to determine whether or not they are competent to carry out practical tasks within the veterinary practice, and identify the underpinning knowledge required by them.

The Occupational Standards are made up of a series of units, each of which is broken down into a number of elements. Although these are likely to be updated shortly, the following text will go through the current standards in detail to ensure you understand how to interpret them and cross-reference them with the student portfolio. Any further changes to the Occupational Standards will not affect how they are used, but merely what evidence the students have to demonstrate to show competence.

For level 2 veterinary nursing there are eight mandatory units that each student must achieve, two of which are common units (CUs), that is, used in other NVQs (Table 2.1).

Table 2.1

Level 2 Veterinary nursing mandatory units

Unit and element	Title
Unit CU2	Monitor health and safety
Element	
CU2.1	Monitor and maintain health, safety and security in the workplace
CU2.2	Maintain good standards of health and safety for self and others
Unit CU5	Develop personal performance and maintain working relationships
Element	
CU5.1	Maintain and develop personal performance
CU5.2	Establish and maintain working relationships with others
Unit VN1	Carry out veterinary reception duties
Element	
VN1.1	Make appointments for clients and their animals
VN1.2	Receive clients and their animals for appointments
VN1.3	Process payments for veterinary services
VN1.4	Maintain examination rooms for use
Unit VN2	Prepare for, and assist with, medical procedures and investigations
Element	
VN2.1	Prepare clinical environments, equipment and materials
VN2.2	Prepare animals for medical procedures and investigations
VN2.3	Assist qualified veterinary staff during medical procedures and investigations
VN3	Provide nursing care to animals
Element	
VN3.1	Administer medication to animals
VN3.2	Administer basic nursing care to animals
VN3.3	Administer emergency first aid to animals
Unit VN4	Care for animals in accommodation
Element	
VN4.1	Prepare accommodation for animals
VN4.2	Monitor the condition of animals in accommodation
VN4.3	Clean accommodation to maintain the health and safety of animals
Unit VN5	Support clients in caring for animals
Element	
VN5.1	Support clients during the provision of veterinary services
VN5.2	Advise clients on the care of animals
VN5.3	Demonstrate the care of animals
VN5.4	Provide veterinary materials to clients
Unit VN6	Admit and discharge animals
Element	
VN6.1	Admit animals for care
VN6.2	Communication with clients regarding the progress of in-patients
VN6.3	Discharge animals from care

Table 2.2

Level 3 Veterinary nursing mandatory units

Unit and element	Title
Unit VN7 Element	Perform laboratory diagnostic tests
VN7.1	Prepare diagnostic test equipment and materials
VN7.2	Prepare animals for diagnostic tests
VN7.3	Collect and preserve samples for diagnostic tests
VN7.4	Carry out diagnostic tests and communicate the results
Unit VN8 Element	Administer veterinary medical nursing to animals
VN8.1	Calculate and administer fluid therapy to animals
VN8.2	Administer specialized medical nursing and treatments to animals
VN8.3	Administer intensive nursing care
Unit VN9	Prepare for diagnostic imaging techniques and conduct radiography on animals
Element	
VN9.1	Prepare diagnostic imaging equipment and materials
VN9.2	Prepare animals for diagnostic imaging techniques
VN9.3	Conduct and provide the results of radiography on animals
Unit VN10 Element	Prepare for veterinary surgical procedures
VN10.1	Prepare surgical environments for veterinary surgical procedures
VN10.2	Select and prepare veterinary surgical equipment and materials
VN10.3	Prepare animals for veterinary surgical procedures
Unit VN11 Element	Assist the veterinary surgeon during surgical procedures
VN11.1	Assist the veterinary surgeon during surgical procedures by providing equipment and materials
VN11.2	Assist the veterinary surgeon to perform surgical procedures on animals
VN11.3	Monitor and assist the recovery of animals after surgical procedures
Unit VN12 Element	Assist the provision of anaesthetics to animals
VN12.1	Prepare anaesthetic equipment and materials
VN12.2	Prepare animals for anaesthesia
VN12.3	Assist in administering and maintaining anaesthetics to animals
VN12.4	Assist in the recovery of animals following anaesthesia
Unit VN13	Manage the availability of resources for the treatment and care of animals
Element	
VN13.1	Manage the supply of veterinary materials
VN13.2	Manage the availability of equipment for use in the veterinary practice

For level 3 there are seven mandatory units that each student must achieve (Table 2.2).

The actual elements within each unit identify the performance, knowledge and evidence requirements that students have to demonstrate to confirm their competence (Table 2.3).

Table 2.3

Performance, knowledge and evidence requirements

Performance criteria	Knowledge and understanding	Scope	Notes
These identify exactly what students must be able to demonstrate practically to their assessor	This states the depth of knowledge students must have and be able to demonstrate, to support their practical ability	The breadth or range of species, conditions, etc.	Whether simulation is appropriate as a means of assessment

Although it is essential for students to be able to demonstrate how to carry out a practical task and be observed doing it correctly and competently, it is also important that they understand the reasons behind why they should do a task in a particular way. For example, we are all told to bend our knees when lifting a heavy object, and the knowledge that we will prevent serious damage to our backs by doing so gives us the information needed to carry out this task safely and competently.

Within most of the VN units and elements, it is not acceptable to use simulation to assess a student. However, first aid is an exception. When faced with a potentially life-threatening case, all will agree that the patient's needs far outweigh those of a student in terms of needing a suitable case for the student portfolio! Emergency situations such as road traffic accidents (RTAs), patients suffering from cardiac arrest, eye enucleations, etc. can all provide essential 'training' whereby students observe their colleagues and assist them during the emergency by holding the patient, preparing equipment, developing radiographs, etc. Having been involved at this level, it is then the assessor's role, at a later date, to generate a suitable simulation of the case. This enables students to demonstrate how to deal with similar situations.

Cross-referencing the Occupational Standards with the portfolio

Cross-referencing involves ensuring that the evidence required by the Occupational Standards and that within the portfolio link together. The portfolio was produced by the RCVS as an assessment tool to help students generate evidence for the veterinary nursing NVQ. However, it is important to remember that the portfolio is only one way for students to provide evidence to meet the Occupational Standards. Guidance notes have been placed at the beginning of each module within the portfolio to help both the student and assessor identify how Occupational Standards can be met by producing evidence of previously observed cases. Assessors should always check with the Occupational Standards that the student is providing sufficient evidence, as in some modules the range of the Occupational Standards for a unit may not be met by the portfolio cases alone. For example, further assessment is essential to ensure that the range of species is met if the student has not had to include a case involving cats, dogs and exotic/small animals. However, if a student is able to meet all the Occupational Standards for a unit with fewer case logs than the guidance notes stipulate, this is fine.

The portfolio is not intended to be the sole assessment tool, and additional observations, questioning, discussions, etc. with students will be required to ensure all of the Occupational Standards are met. The only stipulation is that all of the evidence must be tangible; the assessor should have observed the student and recorded questions and answers along with a summary of any discussion that took place. It is the assessor's duty to ensure that students provide sufficient evidence to meet the Occupational Standards; however the students must also be involved by taking ownership of the evidence that they present and tracking this evidence against the Occupational Standards.

DEVISING AN ASSESSMENT

Trainee assessors will be given examples of documentation to use by their tutors. The forms provided may well differ from the examples included here, but this will not matter as long as they include similar information.

The practical task

When choosing a practical task it is essential to opt for one that is relevant to the level at which the student is studying (i.e. level 2 or 3). Liaise with the student and identify which topics have been covered at college and aspects that need to be covered within the practice to meet both the student's and practice's needs. Having decided on a suitable task, this must then be cross-referenced with the VN Occupational Standards. For simplicity, the following text discusses a task that covers one unit and the three elements associated with it, but it is possible that an assessment will provide evidence across more than one unit or element of the Occupational Standards.

The example assessment that follows is at level 2: a dog is due to come in to have a urine sample collected via cystocentesis (puncture of the abdominal wall with a hollow needle introduced into the urinary bladder to aspirate urine). The assessment will be to 'Prepare for and assist with cystocentesis on a dog'. The relevant unit for this task is level 2 *Unit VN2: Prepare for, and assist with, medical procedures and investigations* (see Table 2.1). The elements that will be covered are: *Element VN2.1 Prepare clinical environments, equipment and materials; Element VN2.2 Prepare animals for medical procedures and investigations* and *VN2.3 Assist qualified veterinary staff during medical procedures and investigations.* You should first turn to the relevant pages in the Occupational Standards and read the 'performance criteria' in the left-hand column for each of the three elements (see Table 2.3). On reading the list of performance criteria (PCs), you should decide which of them you are likely to observe while the student performs the task.

The Element VN2.1 performance criteria include the following:

1. Identify the medical procedure or investigation to be performed and the necessary environmental conditions, equipment and materials.
2. Obtain guidance on the most suitable equipment and materials from qualified veterinary staff.
3. Make sure the clinical environment is clean according to practice requirements.
4. Obtain and prepare the equipment, materials and medication for use in accordance with guidelines.
5. Check that the environmental conditions are suitable for the medical procedure or investigation and the animal's condition.
6. Identify any problems and inform the appropriate person.
7. Observe good aseptic technique and infection control procedures where appropriate.
8. Dispose of surplus and waste materials safely and correctly.
9. Comply with good health and safety practice at all times.

It may not be practical for you to be present for all the preparation. Therefore, in respect of PC3, you may need to ask students how they ensured the clinical environment is clean, etc.; this should provide the necessary evidence assuming the correct answer was given. Similarly, PC6 may not arise if the student does not have any problems with the preparation; in this circumstance you would ask the student to identify what problems might occur in order to cover this PC.

You should go through the other two elements in exactly the same way and identify which PCs can be met during assessment of the practical task.

The 'Knowledge and understanding' column identifies the underpinning knowledge required by the student. The points covered from (a) up to (m) give an indication of the questions that should be posed to the student to ensure the level of their underpinning knowledge.

The 'Scope' column stipulates the breadth or range that must be met. One assessment alone will not ensure all the scope is met and therefore further assessments will need to be carried out and/or questions asked and answered correctly, to enable the scope and the standards to be met in full. These assessments may not require the student to complete a case log for the portfolio.

Having devised the task and identified which performance criteria will be involved, it is strongly recommended that you produce a check-sheet on which you identify which of the PCs are being covered, as in Table 2.4.

Questioning

If you have established that questions need to be asked to ensure that the Occupational Standards are met, these must be written out along with model answers. The purpose of having the model answers is to

Table 2.4	
PC checksheet	
'Prepare for and assist with a cystocentesis on a dog'	**PCs**
Prepare all the necessary equipment and materials to carry out a cystocentesis on a dog	VN2.1: 1, 2, 4, 7
	VN2.2: 1, 2
Ensure the environment is suitable to perform a cystocentesis on a dog	VN2.1: 3, 5, 7,
	VN2.2: 7
Prepare the dog and restrain the patient during the procedure	VN2.2: 1, 2, 3, 5, 7
Provide the equipment and materials as necessary	VN2.3: 1, 2, 4, 5
Monitor the dog during and after the procedure	VN2.3: 3
Record the details of the procedure on the dog's clinical records and hospitalization form	VN2.3: 6, 7
Dispose of any surplus and waste materials	VN2.1: 8
	VN2.3: 7
Comply with health and safety policy at all times	VN2.1: 9
	VN2.2: 4, 7
	VN2.3: 8

demonstrate what benchmark you are making your judgement against. This applies whether the questions are oral or written. These questions, your model answers and the student's answers will each provide evidence for your A1 award demonstrating your ability to plan for the use of different types of evidence and your making judgements based on performance and knowledge evidence. When you write the questions out, make sure you state which of the 'Knowledge and understanding' points they cover in the same way as you did with the practical task. This will ensure you enable your student to meet all the PCs and criteria for knowledge and understanding.

When writing questions where more than one answer is required, ensure you stipulate how many points are necessary, for example: 'State three problems that may occur following cystocentesis on a dog'. Your model answer may include more than three possible answers, including haemorrhage, leakage from the injection site, introduction of infection, damage to other viscera, vomiting if sedation or general anaesthetic is used, but the student will know from the wording of the question that three 'answers' are needed to 'get the question right'. Finally, pay attention to terminology when writing questions. It is recommended that you use terms such as 'state', 'describe', 'list' and 'identify' and avoid using 'how', 'why', 'what', 'where' or 'when'.

Table 2.5 gives some examples of model oral and written questions.

The portfolio case log

Portfolio evidence must be cross-referenced to the Occupational Standards in exactly the same way as the practical task and questions. The completion of a *Module 4a* case log should meet the following PCs:

VN2.1 – 1, 2, 3, 4, 5 and 7

VN2.2 – 1, 2, 3, 5 and 7

VN2.3 – 1, 2, 3, 4, 5 and 7.

Table 2.5

Example oral and written questions

Questions and model answers	Knowledge and understanding
Oral	
1. Name the person you should ask advice from regarding the procedure being carried out and why it is necessary to do so before setting up for the task.	VN2.1 b and c
A. *The vet, to ensure you know exactly what procedure they are intending to perform and what equipment and materials they require so that these can all be got ready beforehand.*	
2. State any changes to the environmental conditions you would make if the patient had been a cat rather than a dog.	VN2.1 d and e
A. *Check all the windows are shut, keep noise to a minimum and ask colleagues not to bring a dog into the room while we carry out the cystocentesis.*	
3. State where you would dispose of the needle and syringe after the vet has finished with them?	VN2.1 h and i
A. *Needle into the sharps bin and the syringe into clinical waste.*	
Written	
1. State 3 problems that may occur following cyctocentesis in a dog.	VN2.1 g
A. *Haemorrhage, leakage from injection site, introduction of infection, damage to other viscera, vomiting if sedation or general anaesthetic were used.*	VN2.2 g VN2.3 e VN2.2 f
2. Describe the action you would take for the three problems you stated in question 1.	
A. *Inform the vet immediately, place an aseptic dressing over any haemorrhage, ensure the dog has a patent airway and clean up any vomit from around its mouth and in the kennel, provide clean bedding as necessary.*	VN2.2 g
3. List 4 potential health and safety risks for the staff involved with carrying out a cystocentesis on a dog.	VN2.1 j VN2.2 h
A. *Injury to back if lifting patient incorrectly, being bitten by the dog, being stabbed by the needle, zoonoses if urine infected with leptospirosis and anaesthetic gases if dog anaesthetized.*	
4. Describe the preventative action you could take to reduce the 4 risks identified in question 3.	VN2.1 h VN2.3 g
A. *Never lift a large dog on your own, if unsure of the dog's temperament put a muzzle on it, keep the patient as still as possible during the procedure and dispose of the needle immediately after use, wear gloves when handling urine.*	

Your assessor tutor will confirm how many assessments you have to undertake and in doing so how many units or elements have to be covered during each individual assessment or overall. Similarly, the tutor will stipulate how many oral and written questions you should devise for each assessment. The A1 award is a national one but the different awarding bodies (e.g. City and Guilds, Edexcel, etc.) may well have slightly different evidence requirements and it is essential that you meet these.

The assessment plan

You should either complete the assessment plan in advance with the student or discuss it once completed and agree the date on which the assessment will take place. You must ensure that students understand what is expected of them in terms of being observed doing a task and what the task is, that questions will be asked of them and that, as in the example task given here, a portfolio case log will need to be completed.

Advise them to look at the relevant Occupational Standards in order for them to determine the level of underpinning knowledge that is expected of them.

An assessment plan should contain the following information:

- the name of the student veterinary nurse and assessor
- the unit(s) and element(s) being assessed
- the date on which the assessment will take place
- the location of the assessment
- the methods of assessment and sources of evidence, e.g.:
    - practical task – observation of the task
    - questioning – student's answers
    - portfolio case log – assessment of the case log
- equipment and materials required
- special assessment requirements
- a date on which the plan was actually agreed with the student
- assessor and student signatures
- postassessment review date.

Box 2.2 is an example assessment plan. Note that the example planning form is just that, and if you are provided with a different style form to complete, or you wish to devise your own, that does not matter.

BOX 2.2 *Example assessment plan*	**Name of student veterinary nurse:** A Student **Name of assessor:** Jill Warner **Unit(s):** VN 2 **Element(s):** VN 2.1, 2.2 and 2.3
	Date on which assessment will take place: 1 April 2005
	Location of assessment: Prep room
	Method of assessment and sources of evidence: ● Practical task/observation of task ● Oral and written questions/student's answers ● Portfolio case log/assessment of case log
	Equipment and materials required: Anne to obtain suitable equipment and materials for the cystocentesis on a dog
	Special assessment requirements: Student being observed by trainee assessor and assessor's tutor and is likely therefore to be more nervous.
	Date assessment plan agreed with student: 28 March 2005
	Student's signature:
	Assessor's signature:
	Post assessment review date: 4 April 2005 to assess portfolio case log

You must ensure the information given to students about the assessment is clear.

The *date* on which the assessment will take place must always be in advance of that on which you agreed the plan itself. In time, once the student is confident with the assessment process, it may be that you both agree to an impromptu assessment as the student may be waiting for a specific case to present itself.

Where the assessment takes place obviously depends on the task itself. If unable to use the prep room because it is too busy or you feel it best to be somewhere quieter for the student's sake, you must ensure that the student is not disadvantaged in anyway and has all the necessary equipment and materials to perform the task under normal working conditions.

With the example assessment in Box 2.2, the student has to obtain guidance on the most suitable *equipment and materials* from qualified veterinary staff (see element VN2.1 PC 2). Therefore it is an evidence requirement that the student asks guidance from their vet as to which equipment and materials they require for the task.

If you are unsure what to include within the *special assessment requirements* box discuss this with your tutor. The A1 award, like all assessment and verification awards, involves assessment and verification of a broad range of NVQ qualifications and includes levels 1 to 5. Some NVQ students (candidates) may have learning difficulties and as an assessor you must demonstrate how you would adapt the assessment to meet the individual needs of your students. When assessing students with varying degrees of dyslexia, hearing impairment and nervousness, it may simply be that you need to allow more time for the assessment itself, provide typewritten questions rather than handwritten ones, or type out the oral questions for the student to read as well as asking them orally. Think how easy it is to forget the question you have just been asked when you are very nervous. Simple things like these help put such students at ease and provide a fair and reliable assessment ensuring they have every opportunity to present sufficient evidence to demonstrate their abilities. Further guidance on special assessment arrangements is given in the next chapter.

The *review* date is always after the assessment has taken place. It may be, as in the example plan, a few days later to give the student time to write up the case log. It may also be several weeks or months later; this allows time for another assessment to ensure the student is still competent either with an identical task or with a similar task (e.g. with a different species).

ASSESSING STUDENTS

When assessing students you must be as unobtrusive as possible. Obviously you need to be in a position to observe the students, but you should stand back and allow them to get on with the task itself. Do not interrupt them during the task even if they get something wrong – unless, of course, it is life threatening to the patient, themselves or colleagues. This policy must also be explained to whomever the students are working alongside, as if others tell your students what to do next this would defeat the object of the assessment. The whole purpose of an assessment is to ascertain students' level of competence. Do not assume that you can ask them the questions as they go along as this may put them off their stride and make them forget to do something they would otherwise have done. If students wish to talk their way through the task that is fine, but they should not feel they have to if this does not come naturally. Students must remember to actually perform the task rather than just explain in great detail what they intend to do, as this part of the assessment is practical. Knowledge and understanding are assessed by questioning.

There is no need to give students the written and oral questions in advance to look at, as in any other form of assessment you do not get to see the 'test' beforehand. However, during the discussion and planning stage of the assessment you should confirm that there will be questions and that students are advised to look at the relevant Occupational Standards relating to the assessment. Within the knowledge and understanding columns are a number of questions that will pinpoint exactly what students need to know to meet the knowledge evidence requirements.

It does not matter in what order students complete the assessment. You may wish to ask them to complete the written questions before the observation and ask the oral ones after. Do what works best for both parties. During the assessment, you can either write down the student's answers to the oral questions or use a highlighter pen and identify on your model answers those given by the student. If a student gives answers that you have not included in your model answers, you can simply write them in. On several occasions when tutoring D32 and D33 in which a vet was the assessor and had written questions and model answers, it was commented that the student had provided different answers to the ones that were expected. The most likely explanation for this discrepancy is that nurses and vets have a slightly different perspective on cases, nurses being likely to think in terms of actually 'nursing a patient' and vets probably more in clinical terms. As long as the answers are correct this does not matter at all.

However, they are recorded, both you as the assessor and the student should sign and date the oral answers to authenticate them. The written answers should also be signed and dated by the student in the same way.

JUDGING EVIDENCE

It is essential that your assessment decisions be based on *all* the evidence presented – that is, on how students performed practically as well as on their knowledge evidence in those assessments where questioning has been part of the assessment process. The Occupational Standards stipulate both the performance and knowledge requirements and your decision must be made on the basis of whether a student has met these or not. Practical assessment and oral questioning is observed and as such it is clear that the evidence is indeed produced by the student. Written evidence can be more difficult to judge, however. Students should always sign and date any written evidence to authenticate it as being their own work and if handwritten it is easier to identify as their own. However, if for any reason you are unsure of the authenticity of a student's evidence, you need to clarify this, as copying directly from script or another student's work is unacceptable. By simply asking the student to explain something in detail verbally to you, should enable you to judge their knowledge on a subject and whether they produced the work. Alternatively you could ask students outright if the evidence is their own. However, careful handling is required in what can potentially be a very sensitive issue.

It may be that you judge a student to be practically competent but whose underpinning knowledge is insufficient to meet the standards, or vice versa. In such cases you would need to confirm this during the feedback stage and arrange for part of the assessment to be reassessed at a mutually agreed date. This is the situation with the RCVS independent assessments; students who fail one multiple choice paper only or do not gain enough marks in one section of the practical exam only have to retake one written paper or do a one-section resit. As a rule, though, any students who are generally weak should do the whole assessment again.

GIVING FEEDBACK

Feedback should come as soon as possible after an assessment. Always be aware of why you are giving feedback – which is to help students improve as well as to confirm what they already do well. You can discuss with the student whether you give feedback immediately after the practical task and before you ask the questions. The student may prefer to complete the assessment without interruption. Or you may wish to say well done, and everything was great, but that you will give more feedback after the questions session.

It is recommended that you ask students how they feel the practical part of the assessment went. If they did well you can be positive and say so, but if they have not done well this enables them to identify any aspects they were unhappy with, or discuss any mistakes, rather than you having to point them all out. Obviously if they made any errors they are unaware of you must enlighten them, but you should do this as constructively as possible. Avoid making feedback into a personal attack. For example, if the dog's hind legs got in the vet's way during the assessment do not say: 'You are not very good at holding dogs'. If instead you ask 'How do you think you could have prevented the dog from kicking the vet?' this enables the student to identify how to do better next time. If a student clearly does not know how to restrain a dog in either sternal or lateral recumbency for this procedure you must explain this and demonstrate it practically as well. This applies to each aspect of the assessment.

Feedback on the students' oral and written answers may well involve your explaining the correct answers and if necessary giving out a copy of your model answers. Alternatively, you may suggest that students go away and research/revise further and then represent their answers at an agreed date and time.

The log sheet

If students have to complete a portfolio case log as part of the assessment, allow them a few days following the practical assessment to do this. You will have discussed how well they have already done and any action to be taken, but as the case log forms part of the overall evidence you will have to explain that you cannot confirm they have met the national standards until you have assessed the case log as well. Once the case log is completed, you need to assess the log sheet, ask questions as necessary and give your student feedback on this too.

Case log 2.1 is an example log sheet of 4a Cystocentesis.

The feedback record

At this stage the 'feedback record' can be signed off by both of you. This may be a specifically designed form, or you may wish to use the assessment planning and tutorial record to record your written feedback. It is good practice to provide some form of written feedback prior to assessing the case log to confirm how the practical task and questioning went. This should be initialled and dated by both you and the student.

Give the student a copy of the signed 'feedback record', which should include the following information:

- the name of the student veterinary nurse
- the unit(s) and element(s) being assessed
- the date on which the assessment took place
- the performance criteria and sources of evidence, e.g.:
  - practical or observation
  - questioning, written/oral
  - portfolio
- confirmation of the assessment decision and feedback
- assessor and student signatures and date of signing.

Figure 2.1 is an example of an individual feedback record, which is included to demonstrate best practice. However, you should check with your assessor tutor whether you need to complete one like this as evidence for your assessor training or whether there is an acceptable alternative.

Finally, you should confirm the next stage with the student. If part of the assessment was excellent, but part resulted in the student not meeting the national standard overall, you need to arrange for another assessment to cover the unmet criteria as necessary. This, for example, may mean a reassessment of only a practical assessment or only the question session.

Case log 2.1 Log sheet 4a – prepare for and assist with medical procedures and investigations

Student veterinary nurse's name:		A Student	VN enrolment no:	E2004
1. Case details:	Species:	Canine	Age:	9 years 3 months
	Breed:	Labrador	Sex:	F entire
			Weight:	32.9 kg
2. Procedure prepared for:			3. Date:	1 April 05

Assessor's comments:

2. Procedure prepared for:

Cystocentesis

4. Preparation of the environment in which the procedure took place:

I checked with the vet who said he wanted to perform the cystocentesis on the prep room table. I then cleaned the table with Trigene at a dilution of 1:20. Our table is electronic and can be raised and lowered. I put the table to its lowest setting so that we would not have to pick the dog up as she is quite heavy. The prep room is kept at a constant temperature and I did not alter this.

5. Preparation of the equipment and materials:

Having checked with the vet, I prepared the following:
electric clippers – checked for broken
teeth, brushed excess hair off and sprayed with Clippercide
Hibiscrub (chlorhexidine) – placed in a bowl with warm water
cotton wool
gauze swabs – sterile pack of five swabs
three-way tap
20 ml syringe
20 g needle × 1½ in
surgical gloves
Boric Acid urine sample pot
plain sterile urine pot
kidney dish.

What dilution of Hibiscrub did you use?
A 1:20 diluted with water

continued overpage

Case log 2.1 – continued

6. Assisting with the procedure: Describe the following briefly;

How the animal was prepared, handled and restrained:

The dog was given a premed of acepromazine and Vetagesic (buprenorphine) subcutaneously 45 minutes beforehand.

She was able to walk to the prep room where she was helped on to the already lowered table. Once on the table this was raised.

Another nurse clipped her abdomen and removed excess hair using a small dust buster. The area was then cleaned with Hibiscrub and cotton wool. Care was taken not to press excessively on her abdomen as we did not want her to urinate before a sample was collected.

I held the dog's head by placing my left arm under her neck and gently pulled the head towards my body. My right arm was placed under the chest to steady it during the procedure. I talked to her throughout to reassure her.

What dose of acp and Vetagesic were given?
A. ACP 0.85 ml and Vetagesic 1.05 ml

What is the advantage of having the dog in a standing position rather than in lateral recumbency?
A. There is less risk of puncturing another organ by mistake.

State if any additional information was necessary in order to assist with the procedure, e.g. previous records, instructions manuals/reference materials:

An external laboratory request form was filled out with client details and I checked with the vet exactly what tests he wanted carried out. He confirmed bacteriology.

Any other details about your role in assisting with the procedure and monitoring of the animal:

The dog was not given an anaesthetic and the sedative was sufficient to keep her calm while the vet carried out the cystocentesis.

The vet collected the sample and placed it in the sterile pot. I placed the used needle in the sharps bin, the cotton wool in general waste, the syringe in clinical waste and the excess urine down the sink.

The dog was put back in her kennel after we checked that there was no evidence of leakage at the site of collection.

If you were unsure of the dog's temperament, what precautions might you have taken?
A. I would have put a muzzle on her.

Student's comments and signature:

Comments:

This is the second time I have assisted during this procedure and I was confident in holding the dog. I realize the importance of making sure all the equipment and materials are ready in advance. As we have several vets at our practice, we always check with them in case they want something different to their colleagues.

Assessor's statement:

The evidence in this log sheet is a true account of the case/procedures described and my involvement therein. The work undertaken in compiling the log is my own.

Student veterinary nurse's signature ....

The procedures and details recorded within this log sheet have been observed by myself /* ~~witness~~ (Witness's name ....) have been carried out correctly and competently. *Please delete as appropriate

Comments:

The vet confirmed that Anne checked beforehand what he required and prepared everything as directed. I observed her holding the dog throughout the procedure and she helped keep the dog still and calm. Further questioning on the type of problems that can occur has confirmed underpinning knowledge.

Assessor's name: ....

Assessor's signature: ....

Date: ....

Assessor's qualification: ....

Figure 2.1 Example of an individual feedback record.

Candidate Name: *A student*   Date of assessment: *1 April 2004*
Unit: *VN 2*
Elements: *VN 2.1, 2.2 and 2.3*

Performance Criteria	Practical	Portfolio	Knowledge and Understanding	Written Questions	Oral Questions
VN2.1		*Portfolio*	VN		
1	✔	✔	a		
2	✔	✔	b		✔
3	✔	✔	c		✔
4	✔	✔	d		✔
5	✔	✔	e		✔
6			f		
7	✔	✔	g	✔	
8	✔		h	✔	✔
9	✔		i		✔
			j	✔	
VN 2.2			VN 2.2		
1		✔	a		
2	✔	✔	b		
3	✔		c		
4	✔	✔	d		
5	✔		e		
6	✔	✔	f	✔	
7			g	✔	
8	✔		h	✔	
	✔	✔	i		
VN 2.3			VN 2.3		
1	✔	✔	a		
2	✔	✔	b		
3	✔	✔	c		
4	✔	✔	d		
5	✔	✔	e	✔	
6	✔		f		
7	✔	✔	g		
8	✔		h		

				Yes	No
Assessment decision: National Standard Met				✔	
National Standard Not Met					

Feedback to candidate:

Excellent practical performance, all the necessary information and equipment for the procedure were ready, dog well restrained and monitored after cystocentesis performed.
Portfolio case log well written, questions correctly answered and confirms national standards have been met. Well done.

Candidate Signature: Assessor Signature:

Date:

CASE STUDIES

You should now read the following three case studies and reflect on the planning and suitability of each assessment, the appropriateness of asking questions while observing the student carry out a task, the content and style of the feedback given and the effect this may have in terms of the current assessment and any future assessments. Discussion notes for each case study are given at the end of this chapter.

First, take a few minutes to reflect on the scenario in Case study 2.1 while looking at element 8.1 from the VN Occupational Standards.

Case study 2.1	**Internal verifier** – qualified for 3 years
Unit 8 element 8.1	**Assessor** – qualified for 3 years
	Student – working towards level 3

The student had recently joined the practice from another TP where she had completed the majority of evidence for the level 3 Occupational Standards using the portfolio case logs only. The assessor used the Occupational Standards to identify which units and elements had already been met and discussed with the student those that remained outstanding. It was agreed to plan an assessment to gain evidence of a fluid therapy case for a cat being administered crystalloid. As the IV was due to come to the practice, a visit was arranged to cover Unit 8 element 8.1 – an assessment of the student calculating and administering fluid therapy to a cat. The visit was arranged for 10.30 am to allow for the veterinary surgeon to carry out ward rounds and the nurses to prepare for the operation list for that day. On arrival, the assessor confirmed with the IV that the practice had sufficient nursing staff to allow her to be an observer rather than be involved in the task itself. This is ideal as it enables the assessor to stand back and see exactly how the student performs rather than be caught up in the actual monitoring or nursing care itself. The paperwork had been prepared in advance and, after talking with the student to confirm the reason for the IV's presence and to ascertain that she was happy to go ahead with the assessment, the assessor agreed to get started. On walking into the prep room it was clear that the operating vet was in the middle of a procedure along with a qualified nurse. Their patient was already anaesthetized on the only available table. The student confirmed that she had asked the vet what fluids the cat required (normal saline) and proceeded to fetch the cat from the kennel. She then handed the cat to the assessor while she calculated the drip rate and collected the fluids, giving set, scissors, i.v. catheter and tape. The student then placed the drip bag and the other equipment on the end of the table, which was still being used for another procedure. She took the outer cover off the fluids and then began to open the giving set. She then inserted the end of the giving set into the bag of fluids. As saline began to pour out of the giving set, the student quickly turned off the flow regulator. By now there was a small puddle of saline at the end of the prep room table, the end of the giving set was hanging off the end of the

continued

Case study continued

table and touching the floor and the assessor announced that, as it was very busy in the prep room, she felt it would be best to stop the assessment at this stage. After replacing the cat in a kennel, all three left to go into another room. The assessor then asked the student how she felt the assessment had gone so far. The student confirmed that she was happy and thought it had gone well. The assessor told the student that in fact she did not consider her to be competent for the following reasons:

- The student should not have brought the cat out of the kennels until she was ready to proceed with the task and that she should not have handed it to the assessor to hold.
- The student should have ensured that she had all the equipment and materials ready before the assessment began.
- The student should have suggested that they all go into another room as the prep room was already being used.
- The flow regulator should have been turned off before the giving set was inserted into the bag of fluids.
- The drip bag should have been hung up on the drip stand and the giving set carefully hooked over the stand to ensure sterility was maintained.
- Although the student did get the calculation right, she should have told the assessor the cat's weight before she began the calculation.

Consider the following points:

1. Comment on the actual choice of assessment for a planned IV observation visit.

2. On realizing that there was no space for the student to set up for fluid therapy, who do you think was responsible for deciding whether the assessment should have been started or should have been carried out elsewhere?

3. Should the assessor have preselected a range of materials for the student?

4. Do you consider it essential that the student explains what she is doing while she is working through a practical task?

5. Consider the action that should be taken if the assessor missed seeing whether the student had actually met one of the performance criteria through her own error (i.e. not overseeing the student properly).

6. On evidence from this case study, state whether you consider the student to have met the Occupational Standards.

7. Comment on the feedback given by the assessor and describe the feedback you consider would have been appropriate to give to the student.

Now look at the Occupational Standards for Unit 2 elements 2.1, 2.2 and 2.3 in Case study 2.2.

Case study 2.2

Unit 2 elements 2.1, 2.2 & 2.3

Assessor – qualified for 2 years
Student – working towards level 2

The student needed to produce evidence to demonstrate his ability to apply a dressing and bandage to a dog for Unit 2. It had been agreed between the student and assessor that the next time a patient came in for a redressing the student would select the materials and apply the bandage.

A dog that had had a dew claw removed surgically from the right fore paw 3 days previously arrived during morning consultations for a checkup and rebandage. The vet took the dog through to the prep room. The student sprayed the table with Trigene, wiped it over and then asked a colleague to help lift the dog on to the table, hold its lead and keep it calm by talking to it while he got the following bandaging materials ready:

- a Melolin dressing
- Soffban
- cotton wool
- conforming bandage
- Vetrap
- scissors.

The student asked his colleague to restrain the dog by holding its head towards their body with their left arm while leaning across the dog's body and holding the right fore leg just behind the elbow.

Assessor: 'How else could the dog be restrained?'

Student: 'By being placed on its left side with both legs extended away from the handler who should then hold the lower legs'.

The student then proceeded to carefully remove the dressing, which he looked at to check if there was any exudate and then placed it in the clinical waste bin.

Assessor: 'Why did you put the dressing in clinical waste rather than ordinary waste?'

Student: 'Because it has blood on it and is therefore considered as clinical waste'.

The vet was then asked to check the wound and requested a light dressing to be applied. The student washed his hands and opened the Melolin ensuring that he touched only the outer non-shiny side of the dressing and cut a small piece to cover the wound.

Assessor: 'Why is it important not to touch the shiny side of the dressing?'

Student: 'In order to keep it sterile as this side is placed against the wound'.

Assessor: 'OK, why don't we place the non-shiny side against the wound?'

Student: 'Because it would stick to the wound if it is bleeding when applied and then when the dressing is removed, it might cause the wound to start bleeding again'.

The student then placed a small piece of cotton wool between each toe. He then proceeded to apply Soffban over the foot and above the hock, having omitted to actually place the Melolin over the wound. The padding was then covered with a conforming bandage, which was again applied distal to proximal. The bandage was then covered with a layer of Vetrap as a protective layer. The student then stated he would be ready to return the dog to its owners together with a plastic boot, which he would ask them to put over the foot whenever they took the dog outside.

continued

Case study continued	*Assessor:* 'You selected all the appropriate materials, made sure the patient was restrained properly and the bandage would have been very good but unfortunately you haven't put the Melolin dressing on so I am afraid that you haven't met the standards with this assessment. I'll get someone else to redo the bandage as the owner is waiting'.

Assessor: 'You selected all the appropriate materials, made sure the patient was restrained properly and the bandage would have been very good but unfortunately you haven't put the Melolin dressing on so I am afraid that you haven't met the standards with this assessment. I'll get someone else to redo the bandage as the owner is waiting'.

Student: 'Oh no, I had it all ready but with you asking questions all the time I forgot to actually apply it!'

Assessor: 'I have noted that you selected it, but as you didn't use it you still haven't met the standards'.

Student: 'But surely the fact it was there and I even told you how I would apply it should count for something?'

Assessor: 'Don't forget this is a practical assessment though, not a theory one'.

Student: 'Why were you asking me questions throughout it then?'

Assessor: 'I need to know that you understand why you are doing something'.

Student: 'OK, but all I am saying is that I think if you hadn't been asking me questions while I was actually in the middle of applying the bandage, I wouldn't have forgotten to use the Melolin'.

Assessor: 'Are you saying you don't agree with my decision?'

Student: 'Well I suppose if you put it like that then yes I am'.

Assessor: 'As you know, you do have the right to appeal against an assessment decision and our appeals policy tells you how to do so, but I suggest we sit down together in the office and go through what has happened today and then decide what to do next. Would that be OK with you?'

Student: 'Alright, I just feel that you put me off my stride and although I appreciate I did forget to apply the dressing, in normal circumstances, someone would have told me and I could have then redone the bandage properly'.

Assessor: 'I understand your point and am sorry if I put you off by asking questions while you were bandaging the foot, but I am only supposed to stop you during the assessment if you do something life threatening to either a human or the patient. Would you prefer it if I ask any questions at the end of the practical task in future?'

Student: 'Yes please, I think I would concentrate better then'.

Assessor: 'OK, in the mean time, I am happy with your underpinning knowledge as this assessment has enabled you to cover the remaining knowledge evidence for this unit. You will need to do another bandage using a dressing and we can plan this for later this week if you like'.

Consider the following:

1. Identify which of the standards have been met in the scenario.

2. Consider how the assessor handled the situation and comment on the outcome.

Finally, look at Case study 2.3.

Case study 2.3

Unit 9 elements 9.1 and 9.2

Tutor for A1 training – D32, 33 and 34 holder
Assessor – working towards A1
Student – working towards level 3

The practice has one qualified assessor and another who is working towards the A1 unit. As part of the trainee assessor's evidence, she needed to be observed by her tutor while assessing one of the practice's student nurses. A level 3 student was due to take her practical examinations in 4 weeks' time and the student and 'assessor' agreed to be observed and assessed, respectively while the student positioned a toy dog for a lateral radiograph of the abdomen, showing collimation and centring details. As the majority of knowledge evidence had already been generated, it was agreed that only a few questions would be asked on this occasion. A date and time were agreed by all three parties. The trainee assessor provided her tutor with copies of the following documentation:

- an assessment plan duly signed and dated by 'assessor' and student
- a copy of the relevant Occupational Standards showing the PCs to be met
- a list of questions and model answers written by the trainee assessor:

1. State when a grid should be used.
2. Identify three types of positioning aids.
3. State the reasons for collimating the X-ray beam.
4. State the distance there should be between the X-ray machine and the person pressing the exposure button.
5. If the patient was a cat, state whether you would have used the same equipment to take a lateral abdominal X-ray.
6. State when a patient should be held manually when taking an X-ray.
7. Identify three faults that can occur in equipment that may affect the quality of the radiograph.
8. State the action you would take in respect of these three faults.

The trainee assessor's model answers were:
1. When the part being X-rayed is over 10 cm thick.
2. Cradle, sandbags, foam wedges, ties, Sellotape.
3. To reduce the risk of scattered radiation.
4. 2 metres.
5. No grid but otherwise the same.
6. Only if the patient's life is at risk by administering either sedation or general anaesthesia or positioning aids.
7. Dirty or scratched intensifying screens, 'developer' not up to temperature, film not replaced in cassette, incorrect choice of film, chemicals out of date in the processor.
8. Clean or replace intensifying screens, make sure 'developer' is up to temperature before processing the radiograph, always replace a new film in a used cassette, check with the vet which film is required, regularly change the chemicals in the 'developer' and make a note of the date on which they are changed.

Just before the assessment began, the trainee assessor confirmed with the student that she was happy to go ahead with the assessment itself and in the

continued

presence of the assessor's tutor. The other members of practice staff had been told that an assessment was taking place in the X-ray room and were asked to interrupt only in the case of an emergency. A note was put on the door to this effect.

The student was told to assume that the patient was a 15 kg collie who was anaesthetized and that another member of staff would be responsible for monitoring the patient. She then proceeded to select the following equipment:

- a large cassette
- a ruler
- a grid
- X-rite tape
- left and right marker
- sandbags and ties
- foam wedges.

The student put the cassette on the X-ray table and then placed the 'dog' in left lateral recumbency with the fore legs pulled cranially, tied in place and secured around the cleats of the table.

Assessor: 'Why have you placed the dog on its left side?'

Student: 'I'm not sure but I know we always do'.

Assessor: 'By routinely placing patients in left lateral recumbency, any vet looking at an X-ray will assume this unless otherwise stated, which helps when reading a radiograph'.

The student went on to extend the hind legs caudally and hold them in place using sandbags. The student measured the depth of abdomen.

Assessor: 'When should a grid be used?'

The student stopped what she was doing.

Student: 'When the area being X-rayed is over 10 cm'.

Assessor: 'OK, so what does this dog measure?'

Student: '11 cm'.

Having already tied the patient's legs, the student then proceeded to untie them and lift the 'dog' carefully off the cassette, which she then placed inside the grid. The 'dog' was then repositioned as before. The student then turned on the X-ray machine in order to be able to use the light beam diaphragm to demonstrate how she would collimate the radiograph.

Assessor: 'What measures have we in place to let everyone know that we are taking an X-ray?'

Again the student stopped what she was doing.

Student: 'We have a red light above the door that comes on as soon as the machine is turned on and we have yellow hazard signs on the door as well'.

Assessor: 'Yes well done, how far away must you stand when actually taking the X-ray?'

Student: '2 metres'.

Assessor: 'Can you tell me where you are collimating and where you would centre the beam'.

continued

Case study continued	**Student:** *'I would go cranially to the 13th rib, caudally to the pubis and to both lateral skin surfaces. I would centre the beam approximately mid abdomen'.* **Assessor:** *'Excellent, well done, you have positioned the dog well, I have a few more questions …'* The trainee assessor went on to give the student feedback: 'I am more than happy with the way you prepared for and positioned the 'dog' for this X-ray. You have answered all my questions correctly – well done. Is there anything you feel unsure of or wish me to go over with you?' **Student:** *'No I don't think so, but I would like to practise positioning for hip dysplasia X-rays if possible'.*

Consider the following:

1. Comment on the planning that went into the assessment in terms of paperwork and facilities.
2. Comment on the use of simulation and state the action that must be taken when using simulation as a means of assessment.
3. Comment on the style of questioning during this assessment.
4. Comment on the feedback given.
5. Decide which Occupational Standards have been met.

KEEPING RECORDS

Having completed the required number of assessments as stipulated by your tutor, you will automatically have generated some of the evidence required for your A1 award. You will also have suitable evidence to keep within the practice to demonstrate to your IV and EV that you are assessing your students appropriately. Each student within the practice should have a file in which you keep copies of all assessment paperwork. More details on keeping records are given in the next chapter.

FREQUENTLY ASKED QUESTIONS AND ANSWERS

Always refer any specific questions relating to your assessor training to your tutor who will be able to advise you on the awarding body requirements for your A1 award. Some general questions are considered below.

❍ *How do I become an assessor?*
● You must be either a qualified vet or veterinary nurse with at least 1 year's postqualification experience before you can start assessor training.

❍ *How long does it take to become an assessor?*
● The award can be achieved in 3 to 6 months although some trainee assessors do take longer.

○ *I already have D32 and D33, do I now have to do A1 training?*

● No. However, you do need to demonstrate that you are assessing your students to the new A1 standards, which can be downloaded from the website: www.empnto.co.uk.

○ *How many students will I be responsible for?*

● As a trainee assessor you should have a maximum of two students to assess. Once qualified, you may have more students and how many you can support will depend on how much time you are allocated at work for your assessor duties. The assessor to student ratio is usually about 1 to 3, but you should discuss this with your internal verifier who will advise you according to your experience, etc.

○ *Does being an assessor take a lot of commitment?*

● Yes, in that you must hold tutorials with your students, observe them during their normal working day, discuss topics and ask them questions, plan suitable assessments for their VN portfolio cases, provide them with feedback and advise them on their progress, etc. However, this should be part of your job as an assessor and you should be given time to carry out your role.

○ *Can I expect a higher salary as an assessor?*

● You will have to negotiate this! Most practices pay for the assessor training itself and your job description should encompass the role of assessor together with your other nursing duties. Being an assessor does carry additional responsibilities and commitments.

○ *Who will support me once I become a qualified assessor?*

● Your TP is affiliated with a VNAC who provide an internal verifier. The IV will support you by answering any queries you and your students have, by observing you assess each year, by verifying your assessment decisions and by giving you feedback. They will also hold assessor workshops where you can discuss ideas and problems with other assessors.

CASE STUDY DISCUSSIONS

Case study 2.1

1. Administering fluid therapy to a patient is not a routine procedure and therefore cannot be guaranteed to occur. When planning assessments, particularly for observation by an internal or external verifier, it is best to choose one that does not depend on a specific species or procedure to arise.

2. The reality of working in a busy practice is that another member of staff may well be using the table you need for the assessment. One could argue that, being level 3, the student should be used to being assessed and could therefore have suggested that they go in another room. However, as it was planned that this assessment be observed

by a visitor, the assessor should have organized for it to be under-taken in a quieter area than the busy prep room in order to ensure that the student had every opportunity to present sufficient evidence to meet the national standard. It is the assessor's responsibility to ensure assessments are fair and reliable and this must be taken into account in the planning stage as well as during the assessment itself.

3. Element 8.1 PC 2 clearly states that the student must select and obtain the appropriate fluids, and also obtain and correctly assemble the equipment and materials. The assessor could have preselected and laid out a range of i.v. catheters, drip bags, giving sets, etc. and asked the student to choose the equipment from the selection. Alternatively, the assessor could have devised the assessment in stages, in which the first stage requires the student to collect and set out the necessary materials and equipment. Either of these adjustments would have saved time and aided the flow of the assessment itself.

4. Students vary in personality and confidence and the decision as to whether they explain what they are doing must be entirely their own. Those who are naturally chatty may well prefer to talk, but being nervous may have an effect on whether a student talks or not. The essential thing the student needs to demonstrate is that she actually meets the performance criteria; explaining how to do some-thing will only demonstrate the underpinning knowledge.

5. By looking at the Occupational Standards, the assessor knows exactly what to expect the student to do in practical terms and must be sure to observe the student at all times so as not to miss a vital stage of the assessment. If she is unsure whether a student did actually do some-thing, a question about this can be asked at the end of the assess-ment itself. For example, if she did not see the student dispose of the stylet or cotton wool she could ask where the student had placed it. Similarly, although the student did not tell the assessor the cat's weight, the assessor could determine whether the calculation was correct or not by looking at the calculation and asking the student to confirm the cat's weight.

6. The student was able to demonstrate her practical competence in respect of PC 1 and 2 and the assessor confirmed the calculation was correct in her feedback to the student. PC 3 was not met as the stu-dent did not correctly assemble the equipment. As the assessment was stopped, the student was unable to demonstrate evidence for the remaining PCs. It would be necessary to look at all other previously generated evidence for this element to determine exactly what evi-dence still remained outstanding.

7. Asking the student how she felt the assessment went was a good way of opening the feedback session as this could have enabled her to identify where she went wrong and led to further discussion. As she replied that she felt everything went well and the assessor did not agree, a positive comment followed by constructive criticism was required. However, the assessor here was very negative and did not pick up on any positive aspects of the assessment. A student does not

have to talk during an assessment itself and therefore, although she did not confirm the cat's weight verbally, this did not affect her ability to calculate the drip rate.

The assessor could have handled the situation very differently. For example, the following discussion may have ensued:

Assessor: '*It's very busy in the prep room and there isn't much room for you to lay out the equipment or set the drip up, so I feel it would be better to stop the assessment for the moment. I suggest it would be better to go into the kennels and set the drip up there*'.

Student: '*Oh OK. I suppose we could also use one of the spare consulting rooms if the kennels are noisy*'.

Assessor: '*Yes, excellent. In terms of environmental conditions, what other benefits would our being in another room have?*'

Student: '*By shutting the door, we could make the room more secure*'.

Assessor: '*Yes, that's quite right. Your calculation was correct and I am happy that you understand how to work out drip rates using a burette. Are there any changes you could suggest in terms of choosing the equipment and materials?*'

Student: '*I thought I would have to choose from equipment you had selected, which is why I didn't get anything ready first*'.

Assessor: '*That is one way, but when you realized nothing was ready, what other action could you have taken regarding the cat?*'

Student: '*I suppose I could have put it back in a kennel, but I gave it to you as I thought it would feel more secure if it were held*'.

Assessor: '*Yes, holding the cat for a few minutes would have been fine, but it might have been better to put it back in a kennel as there was going to be a delay while you got everything set up. If you are happy to continue with the assessment, would you like to get everything set up in the kennels so that I can observe you administering the fluids and monitoring the cat?*'

The discussion confirms that in fact the student does understand what is expected of her and how to present relevant evidence if the circumstances allow. By the assessor suggesting they carry on with the assessment, this positive encouragement should enable the student to go on and present the evidence she requires to meet the Occupational Standards.

Case study 2.2

1. Element	PCs	Knowledge	Scope
VN2.1	1, 2, 3, 4, 7, 8, 9	h, i	A(i), B–, C(i)(v), D(ii)(iii), E(i)dog
VN2.2	1, 2, 3, 4, 5, 7, 8	c	A–, B(i)(v), C(i)dog, D(iii)
VN2.3	1, 2, 4, 5, 7, 8	d, c	A(v), B(i)dog, C(ii)(iii), D–

2. It was clear from the beginning of the assessment that the student had chosen the correct materials and asked for the patient to be suitably restrained. As the student had already selected the Melolin dressing and was preparing to use it before the assessor asked the questions relating to its use, the student was unlikely to have been put off by the questioning technique and the assessor's decision was correct – that is, as the student did not apply the dressing he cannot be considered to have met the Occupational Standards (i.e. to have applied a suitable bandage). The assessor gave clear feedback and explained why the standards had not been met. The discussion that ensued was handled calmly and prevented the situation from becoming confrontational, enabling both assessor and student to work towards the next assessment in a constructive way.

Case study 2.3

1. Excellent planning was demonstrated and all parties involved were consulted. By seeing the paperwork in advance, the tutor was able to determine which A1 elements the trainee assessor had met.

2. As this assessment was purely for the student to gain additional practice in radiography positioning prior to sitting her practical examinations and as a training exercise for the trainee assessor, the use of simulation was appropriate. However, simulation alone would not be an acceptable means of generating evidence for this unit. Simulation must involve the use of all the equipment and materials that would normally be required for a task. Usually live animals should also be used, but for health and safety reasons this was not practical in this case. If unsure about the use of simulation, the trainee assessor should always first check within the Occupational Standards and then contact the IV.

3. Care must be taken to ensure that students are able to carry out the practical task to the best of their ability. Any interruption may put them off their stride and result in their forgetting to do something they would otherwise have done. Assessments have been observed where the student is very experienced and has an excellent working relationship with the assessor and was therefore happy to answer questions while carrying out the assessment task. It can enable discussion and clarification to be sought where a student is unsure of something. However, although you may feel that it is best to talk about something as it arises rather than leave it until the end, any negative comments may have a detrimental affect on the student's performance for the remainder of the task. Ideally, you should know your student well enough to determine the best method to use. It is strongly recommended that you ask individual students at the time whether they would prefer to answer questions during the task or at the end. This demonstrates that you are taking individual needs into consideration and encouraging access to fair and reliable assessment.

4. The trainee assessor gave encouragement throughout the assessment by confirming the student had answered the questions correctly.

There was no need to ask the student how she felt the assessment went as she had clearly demonstrated her competence. However, the 'assessor' encouraged the student to ask for help, which is excellent.

5.
Element	PCs	Knowledge
9.1		c, e, h, k

As this was a simulation, only knowledge and understanding can be assessed for this assessment.

3

The Role of the Assessor in Practice

Essentially, the role of assessors is to assess their students against the veterinary nursing Occupational Standards and decide whether or not they are competent. In addition, assessors must support their students throughout their training by being their mentor, advising them on what evidence to collect, holding tutorials and giving them feedback and encouragement on their progress.

WHAT MAKES A GOOD ASSESSOR?

Assessors are all either veterinary surgeons or listed veterinary nurses. However, they come with various levels of experience and have received assessor training from different sources. This has a bearing on the expectation of the assessment process and the way that different assessors assess their students. Fundamentally, though, all have the same interest at heart, which is to ensure that students have access to fair and reliable assessments and to provide them with as much guidance and support as possible.

Assessment is not about seeing how little a student knows; it should, rather, provide them with an opportunity to demonstrate practically or theoretically (or both) how much they do know. Therefore students must be assessed only when both they and their assessor feel they are ready. Agreeing assessments in advance, albeit on occasion at short notice, prevents the frustration and time lost when clearly a student is not ready to be assessed. That does not mean they will always meet the national standards! In many assessments where students have not been competent, far from being a completely negative experience, those present agreed that at least the practice and student were immediately made aware that additional training/guidance was needed. The skill here lies in the feedback given by assessors to ensure that the students concerned are not demoralized and also are made aware of what they need to do in order to be competent next time.

Many assessors find it hard to know the level to which they should assess the actual contents of their student's case logs. It is vital to assess students only against the VN Occupational Standards for the level at which they are currently studying (i.e. level 2 or level 3). This ensures the credibility of the qualification the students are training towards. Practical assessments and portfolio evidence of students being assessed both below and above the relevant Occupational Standards have been observed, neither of which provides reliable evidence of a student's competence.

Assessors may also feel it reflects badly on them if the case logs are not perfect. However, it is vital to remember whose work the portfolio is and that the wording and presentation are likely to reflect the student's own writing style and experience. The portfolio is an aide mémoire of an observed practical assessment. Detailed guidance on portfolio compilation is given in the next chapter.

> An assessor must:
> - always assess to the relevant National Occupational Standards
> - continue to undertake appropriate CPD, including annual attendance at VNAC meetings
> - be impartial
> - remember whose work it is
> - provide clear and constructive feedback.

TYPES OF ASSESSMENT AND EVIDENCE REQUIREMENTS

There has been a tendency within the veterinary nursing NVQ to assume that the portfolio is the only evidence requirement. However, it is essential to realize that this is only one type of evidence and that, on its own, it will not enable a student to provide sufficient evidence to meet the Occupational Standards for level 2 and 3, respectively. (For further guidance on using the Occupational Standards and cross-referencing them to a practical task, the portfolio and questions, please refer to the previous chapter.)

There are six types of assessment method used within the veterinary nursing NVQ for students to provide evidence of meeting the Occupational Standards. These include:

- observation
- portfolio
- questioning
- simulation
- multiple choice question papers
- practical exams.

There are also diverse means of evidence collection including:

- witness statements
- tape recordings and video footage
- photographs.

Observation

The previous chapter on assessor training discussed the process of planning assessments, making judgements and giving feedback. However, the reality of veterinary practice is that you may not always have time to plan in advance for every assessment you wish to observe. Nursing is a very practical profession and observing students carrying out their role under normal working conditions within their normal working environment is a vital means of assessing their level of competence. Therefore, if a case presents itself unexpectedly, the opportunity should not be missed simply because you and the student have not signed an assessment plan.

If the student and any other staff involved are happy, a verbal agreement at the time will be quite sufficient. The important thing is to assess students against the relevant Occupational Standards, provide them with feedback on how they performed and record this on either the tutorial record or a feedback sheet. Assessor training provides an essential understanding of a process, but once achieved, common sense must prevail and assessments fit the needs of the students and the working environment.

One possible arrangement is planning and agreeing with students in advance to assess a particular case when one presents itself. It may be they are waiting for a particular species or procedure to use as evidence and, although agreed in advance, an actual date and time cannot be specified. The level of experience and confidence of the student will be factors in determining whether it is appropriate to assess at short notice.

Do not limit the number of observed assessments to the number of portfolio case logs. Any practical task that students are expected to undertake must be observed initially to ensure they are competent, again if they did not meet the national standards, or if they did then again at a later date to ensure that they are still competent, or using another species to ensure they can perform the task and demonstrate different handling skills, use different equipment, etc. The Occupational Standards themselves give a clear indication of the type of practical assessments you need to observe the student perform, in the same way as they stipulate the level and type of knowledge and understanding the student must provide evidence for.

Portfolio

Each case being submitted within a student's portfolio must have been observed either by the assessor or by another person acting as a witness or evidence gatherer. Within each module of the portfolio, individual case logs act as an aide mémoire supporting the observed assessments of students, during which they will have demonstrated a variety of monitoring and nursing skills. Assessment includes both the initial observation and assessment of the case log itself. Students should be encouraged to have a copy of the Occupational Standards when writing up case logs to help them identify the evidence requirements needed within portfolio cases and modules.

Portfolio evidence can be initially looked at by the assessor if preferred, but is best assessed during a tutorial session with the student. This arrangement enables feedback to be given, and questions to be asked and written in the margins together with the student's answers. It is not good assessment practice to look at a case log, write questions on it, hand it back to the student to answer and then have it back again to check the answers. This does not allow for discussion or feedback and is very time consuming for all concerned. Discussion between assessor and student is a valuable part of any tutorial session and allows the opportunity for clarification by both parties. Assessors can check a student's underpinning knowledge and a student can be provided with additional theoretical information or explanation. There is further guidance and advice regarding tutorials in the next chapter.

Module summary sheets must be completed for each module by the assessors, who should include a reflective comment on the student's progress while producing evidence for the module. Where more than one assessor has been involved, each can either write individual comments on the same sheet or use a separate summary sheet if preferred. Assessors must also provide an overview for verification purposes of the type of evidence that has been produced to cover the relevant units and elements.

Questioning

Questioning as an assessment method is useful in several respects. First, on completion of a portfolio module, it may be that additional evidence will be required in order to meet the scope of the relevant unit(s) of the Occupational Standards. Questioning is an excellent means of enabling a student to provide such additional evidence to support a portfolio module. Also, underpinning knowledge as well as practical skills must be assessed and the use of oral and written questions will enable students to provide evidence to demonstrate this. Third, questioning can be used during the assessment of portfolio cases as a means of providing clarification, or additional evidence within the portfolio where information has been omitted from the actual text. This often occurs when a student completes the first case log within a new module. However, it is expected that on completing further case logs, the student will naturally include the previously omitted information, although questioning on other aspects of the case is likely to be required.

Unlike in assessor training, where a set number of questions may have to be devised, there is no minimum or maximum limit on the number of questions that need to be asked. The only stipulations are that they are relevant to the assessment and that both questions and answers are recorded. It is not sufficient to write a question and state 'correct answer given' as there is no actual evidence to support this statement; it is essential to provide evidence to support all assessment decisions.

Simulation

Guidance on the use of simulation and as to whether it is a valid means of providing evidence, can be found in section A of the third edition 3 portfolio and within the notes column of each element of the Occupational Standards. The main indications for using simulation would be for health and safety reasons, in first aid situations and to provide supplementary evidence. Simulation is an excellent means for a student to provide additional evidence to supplement previously assessed real cases or where specific clinical skills need to be practised and demonstrated. The January 2002 edition of the Occupational Standards stipulates that simulation is accepted only within the following units/elements:

- CU2 and CU5
- VN1.3 Processing of payments within a charitable organization
- VN3.3 Administering emergency first aid to animals
- VN7.4 Carrying out diagnostic tests and communicating the results.

Where simulation is used to generate performance evidence, it is the responsibility of the assessor to ensure that the simulated task reflects the requirements of a real working situation (i.e. the environment and resources used). If simulation is used as evidence for the portfolio, a note must be made on the case log concerned.

Independent assessments – multiple choice question papers (MCQs)

Students at both level 2 and level 3 have to sit summative multiple choice examinations set by the RCVS. It is a mandatory requirement that students complete a minimum of 60% of their portfolio evidence before applying to sit for either level of examination. There is strong evidence to support the fact that students who have undergone a substantial level of formal assessment in practice are better equipped for the examinations and are therefore more likely to pass.

The level 2 examination comprises two written papers of 90 minutes each. In paper one, students are required to answer questions on either small animal or equine anatomy and physiology; in paper two, the questions are on general veterinary nursing. The multiple choice format requires students to select one correct answer from four possibilities listed a–d. No marks are deducted for unanswered questions or incorrect answers.

The level 3 examination can be taken only by students who have achieved the level 2 award and received their NVQ certificate. The exam comprises two written papers of 90 minutes each. Paper one covers medical nursing, diagnostic aids and radiography; paper two covers anaesthesia, surgical nursing, theatre practice and exotic species. The format is the same as the level 2 exam.

Practical exams

In addition to the two level 3 multiple choice papers, there is a practical examination. This comprises a series of short practical tests on medical nursing, fluid therapy, surgical nursing, anaesthesia, laboratory and diagnostic imaging. Students should demonstrate their ability to perform a range of clinical skills within these tests; the emphasis is on safe practice. Guidance on appeals and mitigating circumstances in respect of independent assessments can be obtained from the RCVS.

OTHER TYPES OF EVIDENCE

The witness statement

A 'witness statement' is a signed statement by a third party, termed an evidence gatherer, which provides further evidence on the student's performance. The evidence gatherer may be another member of the practice team who does not hold a qualification in assessment, but is usually a veterinary surgeon or listed veterinary nurse. The person must agree to this role in advance or at the time the work is observed and should be aware of the relevant occupational standards to be met by the student. The 'witness statement' should be provided on a piece of practice-headed paper or on the reverse of the actual case log, and state the nature of the task observed, the date it was witnessed and include a reflective comment on the student's performance. Merely stating that a student performed a task on a certain date is insufficient as this simply authenticates a case. As the assessor you should then discuss the case with the student and the evidence gatherer, ask the student questions as necessary and then sign the individual case log.

Clients may also be asked to provide evidence to confirm that a student gave them information about their pet or demonstrated how to give medication to their pet. It is helpful if assessors provide clients with a witness statement and ask them to sign it rather than expect them to produce a suitable statement themselves.

The use of tape recordings and video footage

Within other NVQs, these two forms of evidence are used as either an alternative or an additional means of demonstrating students' knowledge and practical skills. In the veterinary nursing field, they could be used as a valid way of recording a question and answer session or a discussion on a specific topic, rather than having to keep written evidence.

Consent must be given by students beforehand as thrusting a microphone or video camera in front of them without warning is likely to be very offputting. The use of a video camera may be considered to be obtrusive by some, but has been used as evidence by a least one VN student and assessor. It is advisable to place the video camera on a stand. If held by hand, this would involve yet another person or the assessor, who is better off observing the student directly rather than behind a lens. Check with your VNAC first to ensure they are able to provide suitable equipment in order to verify the evidence being submitted.

The use of photography

By their very nature, photographs usually only provide evidence of a split second in time. Perhaps one or two photographs could be taken to demonstrate how a student is able to hold a patient, but the practicality of their place as evidence for the VN NVQ is questionable. The assessor would still need to authenticate each picture, permission would have to be given by owners for the use of a picture showing their pet and students would still have to provide written or taped evidence of their underpinning knowledge.

PLANNING ASSESSMENTS

When planning or actually assessing a student, you should always ensure you have a copy of the Occupational Standards with you. By using a highlighter you and the student can then mark off which performance criteria, knowledge evidence and scope have been met and state how they were met. You should encourage students to take responsibility for demonstrating how their evidence meets the Occupational Standards.

As an essential part of your assessor training, you need to provide evidence to demonstrate your understanding of the assessment process. Several of the forms generated for this purpose can actually be rationalized in order to reduce the amount of paperwork produced within the practice. Assessments must still be planned and feedback must be given, but evidence of this can be entered into the student's assessment planning and tutorial record. You might stipulate that a specific assessment is to be undertaken on a specific day; alternatively, a more general comment might be made that the student needs to provide evidence to meet a certain unit or element, and how and by when this evidence needs to be generated. At the next tutorial, you should then review how assessment is going and whether target dates are being met.

Figure 3.1 is an example of some entries in an assessment planning and tutorial record for level 3 and demonstrates the type of detail that is needed. All time spent on tutorials and theory sessions should be noted along with details of the topics covered or discussed. This provides valuable evidence confirming that the assessor is meeting the RCVS requirements for holding tutorials, providing theoretical support, planning assessments and giving feedback. Two alternative means of recording this information are a diary kept by the assessor in which everything is recorded, or a notebook kept by the students who take responsibility for noting down ad hoc discussions as well as times when they practised a specific task or were given additional teaching on a topic, stating what was actually covered. Such entries should be signed each week by the assessor.

Special assessment arrangements

When planning for any assessment, you should remember to take into account any special arrangements that may have to be made to support individual students. Some examples of situations that would need to be taken into account when planning and assessing a student include:

- dyslexia
- colour blindness
- impaired vision
- hearing impairment
- pregnancy
- bereavement
- physical injury, e.g. broken bone, sprain or strain
- illness on the day of assessment
- nervousness or anxiety relating to tests, exams, etc.
- internal or external verification of assessment process.

As an assessor you must ensure a fair and reliable assessment. Students in the circumstances listed above may be unable to produce evidence that reflects their actual ability unless you implement the measures given in Table 3.1, or similar ones.

Figure 3.1 Assessment planning and tutorial record, level 3.

Student veterinary nurse's name: ....

Enrolment no: ....

Date	Issues discussed	Action to be taken	Target or review date	Student's signature	Assessor's signature
30 March 05	Anne requires some more evidence to complete unit 9 element 9.1 – either an endoscopy or ultrasound case. Whichever one comes in first Anne has agreed to use as a portfolio case and she will answer written questions to cover the other piece of equipment. Anne has completed 60% of her portfolio with only 8 cases remaining. Exam entry application duly completed and sent to RCVS.	Jill to advise vets and receptionists to alert Anne and herself as soon as a suitable case is booked in. Jill then to devise written questions to cover outstanding occupational standards.	Next tutorial – 6 April		
1 hour					
1st April	Theory and practical session on anaesthesia – circuits, circuit factors, flow rates, emergencies. Calculations all correctly answered and circuits assembled	More calculations to be set before practical exams in July. Also gowning and gloving up to be practised. Anne wants to try and complete her portfolio by end of April to leave 2 months for revision etc.	May/June	A student	J Warner
1½ hours					
6 April 05	Ultrasound case coming in next week on 12 April – pregnancy confirmation. Anne to prepare equipment and materials for vet and hold the dog for the procedure. As Anne has used an endoscope for Module 9 Maintenance of equipment Case log 9d the evidence has covered unit 10 elements 10.2 so she can cross-reference this to Module 8.	Jill not working on 6th so to discuss with vet and go over elements 9.1 and 9.2 with them. Ask for written statement on Anne's performance. Jill to devise written questions on patient preparation for endoscopy element 10.3 all PCs and 10.1 PCs 1,3 4 and 6. Anne to complete Case log for 20 April.	20 April	A student	J Warner
45 min					

Table 3.1	
Measures to ensure evidence reflects actual student ability	
Dyslexia	Type questions rather than handwrite them Provide access to a computer at work for typing case logs
Colour blindness	Student to provide overlay relating to their own specific colour blindness
Impaired vision	Type questions in larger font
Hearing impairment	Type out instructions and oral questions in addition to giving them verbally
Pregnancy	Simulate radiography positioning Provide seating arrangements if appropriate Ensure access to toilet
Bereavement	Rearrange assessment time and date if necessary
Physical injury e.g. broken bone, sprain or strain	Allow more time to perform a practical task or provide a seat as necessary Rearrange assessment to one the student can perform with their specific injury Undertake originally planned assessment at a later date
Illness on day of assessment	Allow more time or Reschedule if necessary
Nervousness or anxiety relating to tests, exams, etc.	Explain process clearly to student Allow more time if appropriate Hold assessment in a quiet vicinity if appropriate Make other staff aware assessment is being undertaken to minimize any disturbance
Internal and or external verifier present to verify assessment process	Explain presence of visitors and that it is you being observed not the student Carry out the assessment where there is more space to allow for you and the additional visitor(s) to be as unobtrusive as possible

PORTFOLIO COMPILATION

The portfolio is a means of providing essential evidence of a student's observed practical competence for the veterinary nursing NVQ. The portfolio is ultimately students' responsibility but one for which they should receive continued guidance and support from their assessors during its completion. Experienced assessors, are likely to be familiar with the format and evidence requirements but if you are not then ensure you read through all the Occupational Standards and comprehensive guidance notes at the beginning of each module before your students begin writing up cases. Encourage your students to do the same. This will also enable you both to plan evidence collection and to identify evidence that can be cross-referenced with other modules. Nursing one patient can often provide evidence for more than one case log or module.

Having identified a suitable case to use as evidence for their portfolio, it is essential that students let you, or a suitable evidence gatherer, know in advance. This might by necessity be as a patient is brought into the surgery, but it is important to do this as the assessor or evidence gatherer has to make reference to the student's practical performance as well as the contents of each case log. No one can be expected to comment retrospectively. For this reason, it is crucial that each case log is written up and presented for assessment ideally within a fortnight of the date of treatment. This will ensure that all assessments are carried out within a normal working environment and are current. Assessors must write in their questions, their comments and the date by hand at the time of signing each case log. Students' answers can be written in by the assessor at the same time; alternatively, students can write these in themselves if preferred.

Writing up case logs

Students should be encouraged to make notes at the time of nursing or monitoring a particular patient to help when they come to writing up the actual case log. You should also remind them to keep copies of supplementary evidence such as hospitalization charts, admission forms, etc. to ensure they have valuable working documents to support individual cases. In some modules the inclusion of such documents is mandatory. Cases should be written in the first person to confirm that the student actually carried out the monitoring and nursing care therein. Comments such as 'The dog was placed in sternal recumbency' should be avoided as they do not specify who actually performed this action – was it the vet or another nurse? Students need to stipulate exactly what they themselves did.

When writing the first couple of case logs for a new module, students may wish to present a draft copy to you for discussion during their tutorial. However, they should be encouraged to aim to present final copies for assessment. Students should keep a copy of the Occupational Standards beside them while writing a case log, to help them to know what information they should be including in it. They can then make a note of the case reference number on the standards to show where the evidence has been met. The cases should show progression in terms of the student's knowledge, practical involvement and nursing care, medical terminology, etc. Imagining that they are writing the case log for someone who has no understanding of veterinary nursing may help students to present the information in a relevant manner.

If the student has omitted some information, or you wish to clarify something, this can be gleaned during the assessment and feedback of a case log by your asking questions and making a note of both the questions and the student's answers in the margins of the case logs. Questions and discussions on cases are expected as a means of checking a student's underpinning knowledge. Therefore, each case log should include evidence of this. You as assessor must also meet with the student to discuss and provide feedback on the case log and this should take place during a one-to-one tutorial.

When a patient has been nursed by more than one student, it is perfectly acceptable for both students to write a case log demonstrating the monitoring and nursing care carried out by each individual. Care must be taken, however, to ensure that the two individual case logs reflect each student's individual involvement in nursing the patient. Remember that two students cannot give the same medication to a patient at the same time or date, or offer advice to an owner about the same topic at the same time or date. Therefore care must be taken to ensure that each student's case log is valid. Below are three possible examples of such situations:

- in first aid where one student applies a bandage to help stop haemorrhage and monitors the patient's vital measurements while another student is responsible for setting up fluids
- where a patient has been hospitalized for a few days following surgery and one student completes a surgical or anaesthetic case log and another student a medical case log
- where a patient has been hospitalized for several days and requires intensive nursing following major surgery; the case logs should detail the nursing carried out by each and should also include a copy of the hospitalization chart with the input of each student highlighted to show the actual vital measurements, medication and physiotherapy, etc. given.

Where stipulated, expanded case reports are included to enable students to demonstrate their knowledge and understanding of the condition, treatment and nursing management for a specific case. When writing an expanded case report, students should note that there is no point in merely repeating the evidence that is in the case log itself. One method is to write the expanded report first, then write brief bullet points in the case log and, where necessary, cross-reference these to the expanded report. An example is given later in this chapter. Ensure that, as the assessor, you discuss the content of the report with the student, ask any necessary questions and then sign it off as assessed.

The content of case logs must literally reflect the preparation, monitoring and nursing care carried out, but should not include reference to what could have happened or extensive theoretical background information. The style of writing will vary from student to student; however, if you find students writing an essay, you should encourage them to use bullet points and appendices to prevent repetition. Advise students also not to number the pages of their portfolio sequentially but rather within modules (e.g. M1.1, M1.2, M1.3); this will enable additional evidence to be added to a specific module as necessary.

In some modules, the guidance notes stipulate that the assessor, or another suitable witness, must complete the stipulated case logs; in doing so the person is producing a 'witness testimony' to meet the relevant Occupational Standards. Care must be taken particularly where an assessor has more than one student that individual comments made are specific to each student within the portfolio case logs. For example, in module 2, case log 2a the assessor should complete the case log having observed the student working on reception during consultations. The contents of the actual log must reflect the procedures that the student actually dealt with, rather than a general statement of all the various duties that the student might be expected to deal with. In the latter case, the evidence cannot be considered authentic because inadvertently, the assessor has duplicated the evidence for more than one student.

The use of appendices

Rather than repeating information within case logs, or simply copying and pasting information from one log to another, students can produce an appendix, which can be referred to each time a particular procedure arises. The content of the appendix must reflect how a procedure is performed at an individual practice rather than be written 'textbook' style. An appendix is a good basis upon which to build information, for example, when routinely cleaning out kennels after use or for identifying a standard surgical kit (Fig. 3.2). The appendix number can simply be written in the relevant box on each case log. However, you should make sure students do not omit relevant information to specific cases by merely referring to an appendix. If additional instruments were required for an ophthalmic operation these should be recorded on the log sheet together with the reference, for example: 'In addition to a general ophthalmic kit (see Appendix 1) the following instruments were used: iris scissors, chalazion forceps and a Barraquer speculum'. Your student must hand it to you at the same time as the case log as it forms part of the evidence for that case log.

Figure 3.2 Appendix 1 Small animal general surgical and ophthalmic kits.

Small animal general surgical kit

Scalpel handle × 1 suitable for no. 15 blade
Rat-tooth forceps × 1 pair
Dressing forceps × 1 pair
Mayo scissors × 1 pair
Metzenbaum scissors × 1 pair
Allis tissue forceps × 2 pairs
Spencer Wells artery forceps (large) × 4 pairs
Spencer Wells artery forceps (small) × 4 pairs
Gelpi self-retaining retractors × 1 pair
Langenbeck hand-held retractors × 1 pair
Backhaus towel clips × 4
Needles holders – Gillies × 1 pair

Small animal general ophthalmic kit

Small scalpel handle × 1
Eyelid retractors × 1 pair
Microdissecting forceps × 1 pair
Microcorneal forceps × 1 pair
Ophthalmic scissors × 1 pair
Castroviejo needle-holders × 1 pair

If the appendix is being used throughout a module, it must be handed in for assessment with the first case log. All appendices should be signed by the student to authenticate them and by the assessor to demonstrate assessment has taken place.

Students' comments

This box is for the student to include reflective comments about their role and experiences during the nursing and monitoring care of individual patients. They should not restrict themselves to clinical evaluation of the case, but include evidence of self-evaluation where possible, for example: 'I was pleased with the radiographs taken as they were of diagnostic quality. I feel that I carried out this task in a confident and competent manner, although I was disappointed with the collimation, which could have reduced, but I will use this case as a learning experience'. Such comments can provide a real insight into students' personal development during their training.

Cross-referencing cases

Some of the information within case logs can be cross-referenced to other modules. For example a case used for the laboratory and diagnostic aids module may also be used for a medical nursing case. A separate case log will still need to be written for each case but within the medical case log, where it asks for 'diagnostic procedures and tests', the student should simply write 'see lab case no … page …'. It is feasible that one case may provide enough evidence for four or more case logs. For example, a ruptured diaphragm case could involve a student writing up case logs for radiography, fluid therapy, surgical nursing or anaesthesia. (See the example case logs included in this chapter.)

Module summary sheets

These are provided at the end of each module of both level 2 and level 3 of the portfolio and can be used either to record the student's progress during the completion of a module or as a summative document to provide a reflective comment on the student's progress once the module has been completed. Where more than one assessor has been involved with assessing a student, a separate sheet can be used if necessary. For example, if a student moves from one TP to another and is assessed on the same module, it would be appropriate for each assessor to include a comment on the student's performance. In addition, the assessor should identify the type of evidence that has been generated and where additional evidence has been met as in the example included in Figure 3.3.

Tracking students' progress

Keeping track of which case logs have been completed will help both you as the assessor and the student to know which additional cases are needed

Figure 3.3 Example of a completed module summary sheet.

MODULE 2 – VETERINARY NURSE NVQ TRAINING SCHEME		
Module Assessment Summary		
Student veterinary nurse's name:	*A Student*	Enrolment no: *E2004*
NVQ units and elements assessed within this module:	*VN 1, 1.1, 1.2 & 1.3* *VN5 5.1, 5.2, 5.3 & 5.4*	
Assessment method:		
Direct observation: ✔ *see below*	Portfolio task log sheet: ✔	Oral/written questions: ✔ *see below*
Others (give details): *Discussion*		
Examples of other evidence or assessment methods could include witness statements, work products (pharmacy labels, observation charts, client advice, simulation, etc.).		
Assessor's reflective comments on the student's progress during this module in respect of practical skills and underpinning knowledge:		
Anne has made steady progress throughout this module. Her confidence in dealing with the public in general has improved and she shows a knowledgeable and sympathetic approach when talking to owners about their pets over the phone and in person. I am confident in her ability to deal with most situations while working on reception and that if unsure or concerned, Anne will always seek help and guidance from a colleague.		

Evidence has been generated by my:

- observing Anne working on reception on 02.01.04, 16.02.04, 08.03.04
- observing Anne dispensing medication on 12.01.04, 16.02.04
- Guided discussions on euthanasia, ectoparasitic control in the dog and cat, how to respect clients and their relationship with their animals
- asking oral questions to cover the following elements
  - VN1.1 Scope E ii & iii Knowledge & Understanding a, e, f, g, i, k
  - VN1.2 Scope D ii & iv Knowledge & Understanding a, d, e, i, j, k
  - VN1.3 Scope C i, ii & iii Knowledge & Understanding b, c, f, j
  - VN5.1 Scope B v Knowledge & Understanding b, e, g
  - VN5.2 Scope A iii Knowledge & Understanding a, c, e, g
  - VN5.3 Scope C v Knowledge & Understanding d

The evidence to support the above is in the student's training file within the practice.

Please add a continuation sheet if necessary

Student VN's Signature:	Date:	Assessor's Signature:	Date: ....

This form should be used: (1) To give an overall summary of the assessment of all elements of a portfolio module and (2) To give detailed feedback on an element of assessment when required. The Training Practice should keep a copy of this form.

to provide suitable evidence for the portfolio. It is strongly recommended that you use the actual Occupational Standards themselves as a tracking document. This will ensure that vital evidence is not omitted and you can identify where the evidence can be found by adding this information to the standards themselves (e.g. within a specific portfolio module, by questioning, etc.) (Fig. 3.4).

Some practices keep a copy of the tracking document in a prominent place within the practice to let everyone know, should a particular case arise, which particular student needs to be there. If necessary you should put their name next to a specific case on the operations list.

Although the portfolio belongs to the student, it is essential that each assessor is aware of the student's progress to date. The tracking documents in annexe Ei and Eii of the portfolio can be employed and it can be very useful to include the actual species and conditions or types of cases that are required to meet the portfolio guidelines on them. When using these annexes, you should not forget to check the contents of the 'scope' section of the Occupational Standards as well to ensure that students provides evidence to meet all species, conditions, etc.

Keeping a copy of the portfolio

It is a good idea for either the assessor or the student to photocopy the case logs after each one has been assessed. This will reduce the amount of time spent photocopying on completion of the portfolio. Electronic copies are not acceptable, as they will not have the assessor's handwritten comments, signature and any questions on them. Therefore an actual photo-copy will be the only way of ensuring this valuable evidence is kept. The copy should be kept separate from the original. One student was unlucky enough to have her car stolen with both the original and copy inside. Fortunately, they were later found.

ASSESSING PORTFOLIO EVIDENCE

If you have observed the students concerned, you will know when assessing the case log, how they performed the task itself. If it was another member of staff who actually observed them, you must discuss how your students performed and take this into account when assessing the case log.

Where spelling is concerned, it is unacceptable for any medical terminology to be spelled incorrectly. However, simply not liking the way the case has been written is not sufficient reason to make a student rewrite the log itself, as you should remember that the case log is the student's work. Alterations or additions to the text of the portfolio should not be written in by the assessor. If information is omitted or clarification sought, this should be generated during the feedback session where questions are asked, answers recorded and discussion takes place. You must make a comment on each case log relating to the student's practical performance, for example: 'Anne carried out her role in this case confidently and competently. She understood the importance of obtaining an uncontaminated sample

Figure 3.4 Example of an Occupational Standards sheet used as a tracking document.

ELEMENT VN 5.1 SUPPORT CLIENTS DURING THE PROVISION OF VETERINARY SERVICES

Performance criteria	Knowledge and understanding	Scope
You must:	You must know and understand:	This element requires that you:
inform the client of the veterinary services that are available to meet their needs 02.01.04 ✔ *observation & portfolio*	the veterinary services available and the information required by different clients ✔ *questioning 3a scruffy*	A. support the following clients: (i) current clients ✔ *observation 3b* (ii) new clients ✔ *observation 3a*
help the client with the completion of documentation relating to veterinary services 16.02.04 ✔ *observation & portfolio 3a*	the type of help required by different clients in order to complete documents ✔ *questioning 3a & 3b*	
inform the client of any problems that might occur during the provision of veterinary services 16.02.04 ✔ *observation & portfolio 3a scruffy*	the problems that can occur during the provision of veterinary services ✔ *questioning 2c*	B. support clients during the provision of the following veterinary services:
offer physical and emotional assistance to the client during difficult situations 02.01.04 ✔ *observation & portfolio 2c*	the type of physical and emotional assistance to offer to clients ✔ *discussion 2c*	(i) veterinary procedures ✔ *observation 3a × 2* (ii) medication ✔ *observation 3b*
treat the client's relationship with the animal(s) with respect 02.01.04 ✔ *observation & portfolio 2c*	how to respect clients and their relationship with their animals ✔ *discussion 2c*	(iii) counter sales ✔ *observation 2c* (iv) hospitalisation
provide the client with information on how to contact the surgery during critical situations ✔ *observation & portfolio 3a & 3b*	the information provided to clients on how to contact the surgery ✔ *observation 3b*	✔ *observation 3b × 2* (v) euthanasia
comply with health and safety regulations and guidelines at all times 02.01.04 ✔ *observation*	the principles and key points of the relevant health and safety regulations and guidelines ✔ *questioning 2c*	✔ *observation 2c*

of urine. Health and safety regulations were abided by while carrying out the tests'. This confirms that the student was competent, whereas simply writing 'good' or 'well done' does not provide evidence of this.

Assessing calculations often causes assessors difficulty because they feel the student should perform the calculation in exactly the same way they themselves would. Without wishing to be too controversial, this is particularly evident where the assessor is a vet. You should remember that there are several different ways of reaching the same answer; the bottom line is that, so long as the calculation is correct and the student always includes the units (e.g. ml and mg), this should be all right. For example, imagine a dog weighing 18 kg is to be given a Rimadyl injection at a dose rate of 4 mg/kg and there are 50 mg/ml. This can be calculated as follows:

> 4 mg $\times$ 18 kg = 72 mg therefore the dog requires 72 mg
> there are 50 mg per ml, so divide 72 mg by 50 mg = 1.44 ml
> therefore the dog requires 1.44 ml of Rimadyl.

An alternative way to do the same calculation is:

> 4 mg $\times$ 18 kg = 72 mg
> there are 50 mg of Rimadyl in 1 ml, therefore there is 1 mg in
> 1 $\div$ 50 ml = 0.02 ml
> therefore 72 mg are in 72 $\times$ 0.02 ml = 1.44 ml.

A common question is exactly what needs to be included in the case logs for each module. Case logs must reflect the experience of the individual student and, so long as the Occupational Standards are referred to, the information required should be included. The age of students and their personality too may have a bearing on how they present their work. The following example case logs demonstrate their use and cross-referencing of cases in level 2 and level 3 units.

Example case logs

Level 2

Canine Myffy

■ 2b Dispense medication (Case log 3.1).

> This is an example of a poor case log. It was written by a student dispensing medication for the first time. However, when students perform a task for the first time it is not appropriate to assess them as they should have gained some experience before being assessed to determine whether they are yet competent. No one would be expected to sit their driving test on their first lesson. The assessor has had to ask many questions to gain evidence that should have been included within the body of the case log itself. Although one could argue that sufficient evidence has now been generated by assessor questioning, the case log provides an indication of the student's practical performance and, as stipulated, students must not be formally assessed the very first time they undertake a task.

Case log 3.1 Log sheet 2B – Dispensing Medication to Clients

Student veterinary nurse's name:		A Student	VN enrolment no:	E2004
1. Case details:	Species:	Canine	Age:	10yr 5mth
	Breed:	Border collie	Weight:	22 kg
			Sex:	Neutered female

2. Name of drug dispensed (include trade and generic names):

Synulox (amoxicillin/clavulanate)

3. Legal dispensing category and drug classification:

POM
Antibiotic

4. Dose given (include calculations):

Dose:

12.5–25 mg/kg per os q 8–12 h
The vet prescribed the lower dose of 12.5 mg/kg

Dose given (include calculations):

12.5 mg × 22 kg = 275 mg twice daily

The tablets come in 250 mg strength. The vet decided to round the dose down and prescribed 1 tablet twice a day for 4 days.

Assessor comments:

Define POM
A. Prescription-only medicine – can only be prescribed by a vet

State which drug classification Synulox comes under
A. Antibiotic

Define per os and q 8–12 h
A. By mouth every 8–12 hours

How many tablets did you dispense?
A. 8 × 250 mg tablets

For how many days do we usually dispense antibiotics?
A. 5–10 days. Myffy had an injection on the day of the operation making a total of a 5-day course of antibiotics.

continued overpage

Case log 3.1 – continued

5. Reason for administration and route:

The antibiotics were prescribed as a precaution to prevent infection following surgery to remove a mammary tumour.
Oral medication was dispensed to the owner as this route can be easily administered by them.

Can you state the term used when giving medication as a preventative measure?
A. Prophylactic

6. Health and safety, and other dispensing notes to include: (1) A duplicate copy of the dispensing label; (2) Health and safety issues:

I asked the owner if they are allergic to penicillin as they should wear gloves when handling them if they are. I explained that the course of tablets must be finished.

How should unfinished tablets be disposed of?
A. They should be returned to the surgery.

7. Additional advice/instructions given to client: (state how you ensured the client was able to administer the medication/treatment and any other information provided)

I asked the owner if they were able to give tablets to Myffy and they confirmed that they were. They routinely worm her and did not need me to show them how to administer the tablets.

Date of dispensing: 24 April 2004

What action would you have taken if the owner had said they were allergic to penicillin?
A. I would have given them some disposable gloves to wear when handling the tablets.

8. Briefly state the procedure carried out by you, when processing payments for the items dispensed (if applicable):

The tablets had been written on the client's records on the computer, which automatically calculates the cost. The owner paid the bill when Myffy was discharged and our receptionist dealt with the payment, which was by credit card.

Would we charge for these gloves?
A. No, we give these to an owner free of charge.

Student's comments and signature:

Comments:

This was the first time I have been asked to calculate a drug dosage and then dispense the tablets to a client, but I think I managed it well.

The evidence in this log sheet is a true account of the case/procedures described and my involvement therein. The work undertaken in compiling the log is my own.

Student veterinary nurse's signature ....

Assessor's statement:

The procedures and details recorded within this log sheet have been observed by myself/a witness* (witness's name ....)
and have been carried out correctly and competently. *Please delete

Comments:

Considering this was the first time Anne has dispensed medication, she did very well. She calculated the dose rate correctly and her knowledge on the subject is good. She needs to include more information within the actual body of the case log itself next time.

Assessor's signature: ....

Assessor's name: ....

Assessor's qualifications: ....

Date: ....

There is enough evidence in this one case to produce the following Case logs for Myffy.

- 3a Admit animals for veterinary treatment (Case log 3.2).
- 5a Basic animal management and cleaning protocol appendix 2 (Case log 3.3, Fig. 3.5).
- 5c Administration of medication to animals – s.c., i.m. and i.v. routes – reduces number of cases required with three medications to same patient (Case log 3.4).
- 5c Administration of medication to animals – oral (Case log 3.5).
- 3b Discharge animals after veterinary treatment and witness statement (Case log 3.6, Fig. 3.6).
- 2b Dispensing medication to clients (Case log 3.7).
- Witness statement (Fig. 3.6).

Canine Mable

The example case logs provided for this patient, a springer spaniel, are:

- 4a Prepare for and assist with medical procedures and investigations (Case log 3.8)
- 5b Basic first aid and witness statement (Case log 3.9, Fig. 3.7).

Level 3

Feline Oliver

These example case logs demonstrate cross-referencing between modules and units:

- 7a Medical nursing (Case log 3.10)
- 8a Radiography (Case log 3.11)
- 6a Laboratory and diagnostic aids (Case log 3.12)

Canine Bramble

These example Case logs demonstrate how writing in the first person confirms student performance.

- 7b Fluid management (Case log 3.13), written in 'third person'.
- 7b Fluid management (Case log 3.14), written in 'first person'.

Equine cases

This case demonstrates the use of appendices at level 2:

Warmblood Brood Mare Bubbles
- 5a Basic equine management (Case log 3.15).

The following are examples at level 3:

Thoroughbred Dolce
- 7a Medical nursing (Case log 3.16).
- Normal vital signs appendix 4 (Fig. 3.8).

Case log 3.2 Log sheet 3A – Admit Animals for Veterinary Treatment

Student veterinary nurse's name:		A Student	VN enrolment no.:	E2004		
1. Case details:	Species:	Canine	Age:	10yr 5mth	Sex:	Neutered female
	Breed:	Border collie	Weight:	22 kg	Client type:	Current
2. Case number – identification:		Myffy	Assessor's comments:			

3. Reason for admission i.e. procedures:

Myffy was admitted to have a mammary tumour removed.

4. Date and time animal admitted:

23 April 2004

5. Date animal discharged:

24 April 2004

6. Information given to client when admitted:

I asked the client when Myffy had last eaten and she confirmed that she had given her usual meal the evening before and had removed her water bowl at about 7.00 am this morning.

I checked whether Myffy was on any medication – the owner confirmed she is on Metacam, which would be due to be given this evening. I made a note of this on the consent form and confirmed the dose rate.

Owing to Myffy's age, I asked her owner if she would like us to run a preanaesthetic blood test and she agreed to this. I added this procedure to the consent form. I explained that we would only telephone her if one of the results was abnormal, otherwise we would go ahead with the operation and speak to her afterwards.

I asked the owner to confirm the operation she was booking Myffy in for and then gave her the consent form to read through and sign.

I explained that Myffy would be operated on later today and checked we had a contact telephone number. Our policy is to telephone the owner postoperatively to let them know the procedure has finished and their pet is awake and back in the ward/kennel.

Assessor's comments:

If the owner had fed Myffy this morning, what action would you have taken?

A. I would have asked what time she had been fed and how much food she had been given. I would then note this on the consent form and explain to the owner that the operation would have to be performed later in the day. I would then let the operating vet or nurse know that she had been fed.

continued overpage

Case log 3.2 – continued

I explained that we might keep Myffy in overnight but would confirm this depending on how sleepy she is later this afternoon.

7. Action taken by student on admission of the animal:

I took Myffy through to our kennels and weighed her. The weight was the same as on her records and consent form so no amendment was necessary.
I put her in a large kennel and removed her lead, which I labelled with her name and placed on the kennel door.
I made a note on the operation list in the prep room that Myffy had been admitted, wrote her weight on the board and then asked the operating vet what premed she would like me to draw up for her.
I wrote down on the consent form the required premed, but as Myffy was not first on the operating list, I did not draw the medication up until it was going to be administered.

Why did you wait to draw up the premed?
A. It is practice policy not to leave medication lying around for any length of time. If an injection is not given straight away, the syringe is labelled with the pet's name, the date and the name and dose of medication.

Student's comments and signature:

Comments:

I am confident when admitting animals for operations. I realize that owners are likely to be anxious about leaving their pets and feel I am sympathetic to this. If necessary, an owner is invited to come through to the kennels as seeing where they are often makes them feel more at ease.

The evidence in this log sheet is a true account of the case/procedures described and my involvement therein. The work undertaken in compiling the log is my own.

Student veterinary nurse's signature ....

Assessor's statement:

The procedures and details recorded within this log sheet have been observed by myself/~~a witness*~~ (witness's name ....)
and have been carried out correctly and competently. *Please delete

Comments:

Anne is very good when dealing with clients and has a reassuring manner. If unsure, she always checks with a colleague rather than giving out incorrect information. On admitting Myffy, Anne explained about the preanaesthetic blood test, which the owner opted to have.

Assessor's name: ....

Assessor's signature: ....

Date: ....

Assessor's qualifications: ....

Case log 3.3 Log sheet 5A – Basic Animal Management

Student veterinary nurse's name:		A Student	VN enrolment no.:	E2004

1. Case details:	Species:	Canine	Age:	10yr 5mth
	Breed:	Border collie	Weight:	22 kg

2. Case number – identification: BAM 3

				Sex:	Neutered female

3. Reason for hospitalization:

Myffy was admitted this morning to undergo a mammary tumour removal later today. Owning to her age and the size of the tumour, the vet advised the owner that we might keep her in overnight.

4. Type of accommodation and bedding material used, to include (any relevant environmental factors):

On admission, I placed Myffy in one of our shoreline large kennels. This had previously been cleaned with Virkon and lined with newspaper. A clean Vetbed was put on top of the paper and, once in the kennel, Myffy's lead was removed.

5. Accommodation cleaning protocol, to include (type of disinfectant, dilution of, mechanical cleaning procedures, frequency of cleaning and disposal of waste):

See Appendix 2 for Cleaning protocol
Myffy did not urinate or pass faeces in her kennel. Therefore, the Vetbed was not changed during her stay and the kennel cleaned after she went home.
The Vetbed had not been soiled and was therefore placed in the bin to be washed along with other bedding. If there had been urine or faeces on it, the Vetbed would have been put into soak before washing.

Assessor's comments:

What dilution of Trigene was used?
A. For general use 1 to 200

continued overpage

Case log 3.3 – continued

6. Feeding regimen:

23.04.04   Myffy was given no food or water on admission as she was due to have an operation later the same day.
Postoperatively, Myffy was given a small bowl of water at 5.00 pm and at 7.00 pm was given a small quantity of cooked chicken.
24.04.04   Fresh water given at 8.00 am along with 1½ scoops of Dry Hills adult dog food.

Why is no food or water given until the patient is fully conscious?
A. To prevent vomiting or asphyxiation.

7. Nursing care and monitoring of the animal: Please give details of grooming, wound management, cleaning, monitoring of vital signs and 'TLC'.

23.04.04
The endotracheal tube was removed by the surgical nurse before Myffy was brought back through to the kennels. I then placed her back in her kennel and monitored her temperature, pulse and respiratory rate during her recovery.
The wound was cleaned postoperatively by the surgical nurse. A Primapore dressing was placed over the wound to keep it clean and to help prevent interference to the wound itself and the sutures.
I checked the dressing to ensure that there was no evidence of the wound bleeding. The dressing remained clean and dry.
At 4.30 pm I took Myffy outside on a lead to see if she wanted to pass urine or faeces. She passed some urine – I wrote this on her kennel records.

24.04.04
I took Myffy's temperature, checked her dressing for signs of bleeding or swelling.
I took her outside to urinate, which she did.
I brushed her coat with a soft brush and checked her eyes and ears to make sure they were clean.

Date(s) specify duration of hospitalization 23 and 24 April 2004

8. Medication administered: (details can be cross-referenced to Log 5c)

23.04.04   I administered Myffy's premedication, antibiotics and analgesia by injection. Please refer to Case 5c Myffy
24.04.04   I administered a synulox antibiotic tablet – please refer to Case 5c Myffy

Student's comments, to include: the part the student has played in this case:

Comments:

I feel I gained a lot of experience nursing Myffy as I was able to follow the case through from admission to discharge. I was particularly pleased that I was able to administer all her medications including the intravenous Rimadyl as this would normally have been given by the surgical nurse and not the kennel nurse.

Copy of hospitalization record attached YES ☐ NO ✓

The evidence in this log sheet is a true account of the case/procedures described and my involvement therein. The work undertaken in compiling the log is my own.

Student veterinary nurse's signature ....

Assessor's statement:

The procedures and details recorded within this log sheet have been observed by myself/~~a witness*~~ (witness's name............................) and have been carried out correctly and competently. *Please delete

Comments:

Anne was very caring when nursing Myffy making sure she was comfortable during her stay. When the owner telephoned, Anne reassured her and explained that we wanted to keep her in owing to her age.

Assessor's signature: .... Assessor's name: ....

Assessor's qualifications: .... Date: ....

Figure 3.5 Appendix 2 Cleaning protocol.

CLEANING PROTOCOL – KENNELS

1. Put on plastic apron and gloves
2. Remove patient to a clean kennel
3. Remove bedding and place in wash bin. If soiled, soak in Trigene 1:50 before washing.
4. Remove newspaper and if soiled place in clinical waste.
5. Remove any hair, etc. using a dustpan and brush.
6. Spray kennel ceiling, walls, floor and door with Trigene.
7. Using a cloth or paper towel, wipe the kennel starting with the ceiling and working down to the walls, floor and doors.
8. Rinse the kennel with warm water.
9. Dry the kennel before placing clean newspaper and vetbed on the floor

Dilution rates:
For general cleaning dilute Trigene at a rate of 1 to 200
For intermediate risks use a dilution rate of 1 to 100
High risk areas use 1 to 50

For use in the consulting room and prep-room we use a dilution rate of 1 to 150.

Why is it necessary to brush the kennel out before using Trigene?
A. To remove organic matter as this would prevent the Trigene from working.

Why is it necessary to wear gloves when cleaning kennels?
A. To prevent the risk of zoonoses from handling urine, faeces and hair and to prevent skin contact with cleaning chemicals, which can cause skin allergies, rashes, etc.

Signed by:
A Student
The Assessor
28 April 2004

Figure 3.6 Myffy witness statement for Case logs 2b and 3b.

ALL CREATURES VETERINARY CLINIC

I observed Anne discharging Myffy, a border collie, to her owner on 24 April 04. She gave clear instructions to the client about exercise and feeding postoperatively. I checked her calculation, which was correct, and she then dispensed the medication correctly, again giving clear instructions. Anne checked that the owner was able to administer tablets.
She then made the appointment for a postoperative check-up before giving Myffy back to her owner.

Another veterinary nurse VN D32,33   27 April 2004
Another veterinary nurse

Case log 3.4 Log sheet 5C – Administration of Medication to Animals

Student veterinary nurse's name:	A Student	VN enrolment no.:	E2004

1. Case details:	Breed:	Border collie	Weight:	22 kg	Sex:	Neutered female
	Species:	Canine	Age:	10yr 5mth		

2. Case number – identification:	No. 2	3. Date administered:	23 April 04

4. Name of medication administered, to include trade and generic names and classification and drug form: e.g. antibiotic/cream, sedative/injection, etc.

1. Acepromazine maleate POM sedative injection subcutaneously (s.c.)
2. Vetergesic (buprenorphine) POM opiod analgesic injection subcutaneously (s.c.)
3. Synulox (amoxicillin/clavulanate) POM antibiotic injection intramuscularly (i.m.)
4. Rimadyl (carprofen) POM non-steroidal anti-inflammatory (NSAID) analgesic injection intravenously (i.v.)

5. Dose details

Dose rate:

1. ACP 0.025 ml/kg s.c.
2. Vetergesic 0.023 ml/kg s.c.
3. Synulox i.m. 8.75 mg/kg
4. Rimadyl i.v. 4 mg/kg

Dose given (including calculation):

1. 0.025 ml × 22 kg = 0.55 ml
2. 0.023 ml × 22 kg = 0.50 ml
3. 8.75 mg × 22 kg = 193 mg 175 mg/ml 193 ÷ 175 = 1.1ml rounded down to 1 ml
4. 4 mg × 22 kg = 88 mg 50 mg/ml 88 ÷ 50 = 1.76 ml rounded up to 1.8 ml

Assessor's comments:

continued overpage

Case log 3.4 – continued

6. Reason for administration, basic effect of the drug and how it was administered:

1. ACP &

2. Vetergesic were administered as a premedicant and provided moderate sedation. Both were given by subcutaneous injection. I held Myffy myself and pulled up a tent of skin between Myffy's shoulder blades and inserted the barrel of the needle into the V. I pulled back on the syringe to ensure there was no blood and gently injected. I rubbed the injection site afterwards.

3. Synulox was administered preoperatively in order for the antibiotic to be able to take effect prior to surgery. I asked a colleague to restrain Myffy gently around her neck to prevent her turning around while I gave the injection into her quadriceps muscle in her hind leg. I held her leg and felt in front of her femur for the muscle. I gently inserted the needle, pulled back to make sure I had not gone into a blood vessel and then injected the Synulox. Again I rubbed the injection site afterwards.

4. Rimadyl was administered during the operation to provide pain relief during recovery from surgery. An indwelling catheter was already inserted into Myffy's cephalic vein. As Myffy was lying in ventrodorsal position, I asked a colleague to hold Myffy's leg for me to gain access to the catheter. I wiped the bung with spirit to ensure it was clean, inserted the needle into the bung/catheter and pulled back to ensure the catheter was still patent. I then injected slowly into the catheter.

7. Health and safety issues and precautions taken: *If a controlled drug, specify the recording and storage requirements and attach a copy of the register entry if applicable.*

- Care must be taken when administering medication to ensure the safety of the patient, the handler and the administrator.
- When injections are drawn up it is essential to cover the needle straight away. Under no circumstances must anyone walk about with an uncovered/protected needle.
- On administering the injection the patient must be properly restrained to prevent injury to the administrator. Depending on the route, another member of staff may be necessary.
- After use, needles must be placed in the sharps bin and the syringe in the clinical waste.
- The patient must be monitored for any adverse reaction following administration of medications.

When I administered the above injections, I was happy to hold Myffy for the subcutaneous injection, as she is known to be docile. Intramuscular injections can be painful and I therefore asked a colleague to hold her while I gave this. The intravenous injection was given while she was still under the anaesthetic.

Student's comments and signature:

Comments:

I have regularly administered injections by subcutaneous and intramuscular routes and feel confident with calculating dose rates. This is the second time I have given an intravenous injection and found it straightforward.

The evidence in this log sheet is a true account of the case/procedures described and my involvement therein. The work undertaken in compiling the log is my own.

Student veterinary nurse's signature: ....

Assessor's statement:

The procedures and details recorded within this log sheet have been observed by myself/~~a witness~~* (witness's name...........................) and have been carried out correctly and competently. *Please delete

Comments:

Anne understands the health and safety implications when administering medications and I am happy with her ability to calculate dose rates. I observed her administer each of these injections and she was very competent.

Assessor's signature: .... Assessor's name: ....

Assessor's qualifications: .... Date: ....

Case log 3.5 Log sheet 5C – Administration of Medication to Animals

Student veterinary nurse's name:		A Student		VN enrolment no.:	E2004
1. Case details:	Species:	Border collie	Weight:	22 kg	
	Breed:	Canine	Age:	10yr 5mth	Sex: *Female Neutered*
2. Case number – identification:		No. 3		3. Date administered:	24 April 04

4. Name of medication administered, to include trade and generic names and classification and drug form: e.g. antibiotic/cream, sedative/injection etc.

Synulox (amoxicillin/clavulanate) antibiotic prescription-only medicine (POM)

5. Dose details

Dose rate:

12.5–25 mg/kg per os q 8–12 h (by mouth every 8–12 hours)
The vet prescribed the lower dose of 12.5 mg/kg

Dose given (include calculations):

12.5 mg × 22 kg = 275 mg twice daily
The tablets come in 250 mg strength and the vet prescribed 1 tablet twice a day for 4 days.

6. Reason for administration, basic effect of the drug and how it was administered:

By mouth – I held Myffy's head in a slightly elevated position, gently pulled her upper jaw with my left hand and used my right hand to pull downwards on her lower jaw. Once opened, I placed the tablet at the back of her mouth on her tongue and immediately closed her mouth holding it shut with my hand. I then gently massaged her throat to encourage her to swallow, which she did.

Please also refer to Case 2b Myffy

Assessor's comments:

How many milligrams would be required if a dose rate of 25 mg per kg were prescribed?
A. 25 mg × 22 kg = 550 mg
How many tablets would you have given?
A. The dog would have required 2.2 tablets so I would have checked with the vet and probably given two tablets.

7. Health and safety issues and precautions taken: *If a controlled drug, specify the recording and storage requirements and attach a copy of the register entry if applicable.*

Please refer to Case 2b Myffy.

Student's comments and signature:

Comments:

It was both rewarding and interesting to be able to be involved with Myffy from admission, administering her medications and to finally discharging her back to her owner. I feel I administered the tablet correctly but am aware that if she had been a fractious animal, I may have been unable to have done so without the aid of a pill giver or may have had to give it in food.

The evidence in this log sheet is a true account of the case/procedures described and my involvement therein. The work undertaken in compiling the log is my own.

Student veterinary nurse's signature: ....

Assessor's statement:

The procedures and details recorded within this log sheet have been observed by myself/~~a witness~~* (witness's name ....)
and have been carried out correctly and competently. *Please delete

Comments:

Anne has demonstrated her ability to administer the tablets correctly and safely. We discussed the alternative ways of administering medication and Anne was fully aware of the risks both to the patient and to herself.

Assessor's signature: ....   Assessor's name: ....

Assessor's qualifications: ....   Date: ....

Case log 3.6 Log sheet 3B – Discharge Animals after Veterinary Treatment

Student veterinary nurse's name:	A Student		VN enrolment no.:		E2004	
1. Case details:	Species:	Canine	Age:	10yr 5mth	Sex:	Female Neutered
	Breed:	Border collie	Weight:	22 kg	Client Type	Current

2. Case number – identification:

3. Veterinary procedure carried out:

Mammmary tumour removal

4. Date and time animal discharged:	24 April 04 @ 2 pm	5. Date and time of next appointment:	27 April 04 @ 3.40 pm

6. Describe any preparation of the animal prior to discharge:

Myffy was taken outside during the day to pass urine and faeces. I checked on her hospitalization sheet that she had passed both.
I checked her wound to make sure the sutures were in place and that there was no bleeding, swelling or discharge.
I administered 1 × 250 mg Synulox tablet by mouth and then gave her food and water. As Myffy is normally fed in the evening by her owner, I did not give the Metacam as this would be given later today.

7. Information and advice given to the client:

I advised that Myffy have only lead exercise until her postop check on 27 April to prevent unnecessary strain on her stitches.
I explained that Myffy had been given 1 × 250 mg Synulox tablet this morning and some food and that she was to have a further 1 tablet this evening.
Food wise, Myffy could have her normal diet and to continue with the Metacam as before.
I showed Myffy's owner the wound/dressing and explained about looking for swelling, discharge/bleeding, etc. and to contact us if she was worried at all.

Assessor's comments:

If Myffy had not passed any urine during the day, what action would you have taken?
A. I would make a note on the kennel records. If necessary, I would inform the vet.

What type of healing is achieved by suturing a wound?
A. First intention.

How long are sutures usually left in for?
A. About 10 days.

8. State any medication or treatment (s) supplied to owner:*

YES ✔   NO ☐

Comments:

Synulox (amoxicillin/clavulanate) 250 mg tablets. 1 tablet twice daily for 4 days

*Details can be cross-referenced to dispensing logs
Please see Case log 2b Myffy*

9. Was the method for administrating any medication or treatment(s) to the animal demonstrated to the owner?

YES ☐   NO ✔

Comments:

The owner confirmed that she was able to administer tablets to Myffy.

Student's comments and signature:

Comments:

Myffy stayed in overnight as she was still quite sleepy postoperatively. This was merely a precaution because of her age. I explained to her owner about checking the wound and dispensed the medication. It is our policy to speak to the owners before bringing out their pet. In addition we give a postoperative sheet, which provides the same details as those given verbally. An appointment was made for a 3-day postop check.

The evidence in this log sheet is a true account of the case/procedures described and my involvement therein. The work undertaken in compiling the log is my own.

Student veterinary nurse's signature ....

Assessor's statement:

The procedures and details recorded within this log sheet have been observed by ~~myself~~/a witness* (witness's name: *Another Nurse*) and have been carried out correctly and competently. *Please delete

Comments:

Anne clearly provided Myffy's owner with information about the medication, checking the wound and exercise. She answered the questions clearly and made an appointment at a time to suit the owner.

Assessor's signature: ....   Assessor's name: ....

Assessor's qualifications: ....   Date: ....

Case log 3.7 Log sheet 2B – Dispensing Medication to Clients

Student veterinary nurse's name:		A Student		VN enrolment no:	E2004
1. Case details:	Species:	Canine		Age:	10yr 5mth
	Breed:	Border collie		Weight:	22 kg
				Sex:	Neutered female

2. Name of drug dispensed (include trade and generic names):

Synulox (amoxicillin/clavulanate)

3. Legal dispensing category and drug classification:

Prescription-only medicine POM
Antibiotic

4. Dose given (include calculations):

Dose:

12.5–25 mg/kg per os q 8–12 h (by mouth every 8–12 hours)
The vet prescribed the lower dose of 12.5 mg/kg

Dose given (include calculations):

12.5 mg × 22 kg = 275 mg twice daily

The tablets come in 250 mg strength and the vet prescribed 1 tablet twice a day for 4 days. Myffy had an injection on the day of the operation making a total of a 5-day course of antibiotics. As the tablets were being given as a precautionary measure, the vet confirmed that he was happy to use the lower dose.

I dispensed 8 × 250 mg tablets

Assessor comments:

5. Reason for administration and route:

The antibiotics were prescribed as a precaution to prevent infection following surgery to remove a mammary tumour.
Oral medication was dispensed to the owners as this route can be easily administered by them.

6. Health and safety, and other dispensing notes to include: (1) A duplicate copy of the dispensing label. (2) Health and safety issues:

I asked the owners if they are allergic to penicillin as they should wear gloves when handling them if they are. I explained that the course of tablets must be finished.

All Creatures Veterinary Clinic
43 The Lawns, London SW1 8PS

24.04.04
For ~~Mrs Bogs'~~ dog Myffy
~~8 The Ham, London SW1 3PT~~
8 × 250 mg Synulox tablets
Give one tablet twice a day

Keep Out of Reach of Children
For Animal Treatment Only

7. Additional advice/instructions given to client: (state how you ensured the client was able to administer the medication/treatment and any other information provided)

I asked the owners if they were able to give tablets to Myffy and they confirmed that they were. They routinely warm her and did not need to me show them how to administer the tablets.

Date of dispensing: 24th April 2004

What action would you have taken if the owner had said they were allergic to penicillin?
A. I would have given them some disposable gloves to wear when handling the tablets.

Would we charge for these gloves?
A. No, we give these to an owner free of charge.

continued overpage

Case log 3.7 – continued

8. Briefly state the procedure carried out by you, when processing payments for the items dispensed (if applicable):

The tablets had been written on the client's records on the computer, which automatically calculates the cost. The owner paid their bill when Myffy was discharged and our receptionist dealt with the payment, which was by credit card.

Student's comments and signature:

Comments:

I regularly calculate medication dose rates and always check with the prescribing vet before putting the tablets up.

The evidence in this log sheet is a true account of the case/procedures described and my involvement therein. The work undertaken in compiling the log is my own.

Student veterinary nurse's signature ....

Assessor's statement:

The procedures and details recorded within this log sheet have been observed by ~~myself~~/a witness* (Witness's name: *Another Nurse*) and have been carried out correctly and competently. *Please delete

Comments:

Anne is very vigilant in checking her calculations with a qualified member of staff and always speaks to the dispensing vet if unsure or to confirm dose rates where necessary. Anne correctly calculated the dose rate and dispensed the tablets in this case.

Assessor's signature: .... Assessor's name: ....

Assessor's qualifications: .... Date: ....

Case log 3.8 Log sheet 4A – Prepare for and Assist with Medical Procedures and Investigations

Student veterinary nurse's name:		A Student		VN enrolment no:	E2004
1. Case details:	Species:	Canine		Age:	12yrs 2ths
	Breed:	Springer spaniel		Weight:	15.9 kg
					Sex: F (N)

2. Procedure prepared for:

Fluid therapy – the vet decided to administer Haemaccel.

3. Date: 15 March 05

Assessor's comments:

4. Preparation of the environment in which the procedure took place:

The dog was in a collapsed state and the vet decided to place her directly in a large walk in kennel. This was previously cleaned using Trigene (1:50) and lined with newspaper and a large Vetbed. A heat pad was placed under the Vetbed.
The kennel area is maintained at an ambient temperature of 20°C. Heat pads are available for warming patients and fans for cooling them down.

Is Haemaccel a colloid or crystalloid?
A. Colloid.

5. Preparation of the equipment and materials:

- 500 ml of Haemaccel – expiry date checked, warmed to body temperature
- Giving set – sterility checked
- Swab with Hibiscrub (1:20)
- Swab with spirit
- Clippers – hair removed by brushing, sprayed with Clippercide
- Micropore
- 20 g × 1.25 inch catheter – sterility checked
- Bandaging material; Softban and Vetrap

I removed the outer package of the fluid bag and then broke the seal to the giving port. The giving set bag was opened and the giving set regulator was closed. I then inserted the giving set into the fluid bag making sure I didn't contaminate any part of the set. I squeezed the drip chamber until it was half full and then opened the regulator to allow the fluid to fill up the giving set tubing. I ran it through to ensure that no air bubbles were present in the tubing.
I then hung the giving set up over the drip stand to prevent contamination.

Why is a bandage placed over the catheter and giving set/line?
A. To prevent interference by the dog.

When would you consider the fluids unsuitable for use?
A. If they are out of date, cloudy or had been contaminated in any way.

continued overpage

Case log 3.8 – continued

6. Assisting with the procedure. Describe the following briefly:

How the animal was prepared, handled and restrained.

Manual restraint was used but, as the dog was collapsed, it was only necessary to gently hold her head to one side.

The dog's right fore leg was clipped to enable a catheter to be inserted into the cephalic vein. The skin was wiped with Hibiscrub and then sprayed with surgical spirit. The leg was supported in my right hand and my thumb used to raise the vein. Once the vet had inserted the catheter and blood was evident in the catheter barrel, I released pressure on the vein but continued to hold the leg until the catheter was secured in place using Micropore and the giving set attached. The vet then placed a layer of Soffban covered with Vetwrap over the leg and around the catheter sight.

State if any additional information was necessary in order to assist with the procedure, e.g. previous records, instructions manuals/reference materials.

The vet accessed the dog's clinical records to check her weight before a drip rate was calculated.

Any other details about your role in assisting with the procedure and monitoring of the animal.

I was responsible for monitoring the dog's pulse, respiration, capillary refill time and body temperature while the drip was running.
Please see Case log 5b FA 2 for Mable's vital signs and normal ranges.

In addition to monitoring these vital measurements, what else should you check?
A. Urine output.

Student's comments and signature:

Comments:

I always check with the vet which fluids they require although I usually predict the correct fluids and I am confident in selecting the appropriate items as I have helped with administering fluid therapy on several occasions.

The evidence in this log sheet is a true account of the case/procedures described and my involvement therein. The work undertaken in compiling the log is my own.

Student veterinary nurse's signature ....

Assessor's statement:

The procedures and details recorded within this log sheet have been observed by myself/a witness* (witness's name A Vet ....) and have been carried out correctly and competently. *Please delete as appropriate

Comments:

I have discussed this case with A Vet and he has confirmed that Anne correctly selected and prepared the necessary equipment. She held the dog appropriately and raised the vein. She monitored the dog and recorded her temperature, pulse, respiration and CRT while the drip was being administered.

Assessor's signature: ....

Assessor's qualifications: ....

Assessor's name: ....

Date: ....

Figure 3.7 Mable witness statement.

ALL CREATURES VETERINARY CLINIC

An elderly springer spaniel was brought in by its owner on the 15 March 04, in a collapsed state. Anne helped me place Mable in a kennel and prepared all the necessary equipment to administer fluids to her. She raised the vein and monitored her while the fluids were administered. I am happy with the way Anne carried out these tasks.

20 March 2004

A Vet MRCVS D32,33
A Veterinary Surgeon

Case log 3.9 Log sheet 5B – Basic First Aid

Student veterinary nurse's name:		A Student	VN enrolment no:	E2004
1. Case details:	Species:	Canine	Age:	12yr 2mths
	Breed:	Springer spaniel	Weight:	15.9 kg
			Sex:	F (N)

2. Case no. – identification: FA 2

3. History:

The owner telephoned the surgery at 5.35 pm saying she came home to find her dog had collapsed outside in the garden.

4. Clinical evaluation of patient:

- Mable had a subnormal temperature of 36.7°C (normal range is 38.3–38.7°C) her extremities were cold when touched.
- Respiratory rate was increased to 45 per minute (normal range is 10–30)
- Her pulse rate was rapid at 180 but was weak (normal range is 60–180); the larger the animal the slower the respiratory rate
- Her mucous membranes were pale and the capillary refill time (CRT) was 3 seconds (normal range <2 seconds)

The vet diagnosed that she was suffering from hypothermia (reduced body temperature) and shock.

5. First aid emergency procedure carried out:

On admittance, Mable was put straight into a large walk in kennel and placed on Vetbed with a heat pad underneath and covered in a blanket to keep her warm.
I was asked to prepare intravenous fluids – 500 ml of Haemaccel
Please see Case 4a for preparation of the equipment and materials. It was intended that by giving warmed Haemaccel this would help raise Mable's body temperature and help counteract shock.

Assessor's comments:

Anne and I discussed terms and causes of raised and decreased TPR and CRT.

She was able to tell me that a raised temp would indicate:

Infection, pain or heat stroke and a subnormal one: shock or impending parturition. A raised pulse rate: exercise, fever or pain and a decreased respiratory rate: unconsciousness or anaesthesia.

A raised respiratory rate = trachypnoea: exercise, pain or heat and a decreased respiratory rate bradypnoea: sleep or poisoning with narcotics.

6. Monitoring of the animal:

I was responsible for monitoring Mable's vital signs while she was on the drip. This included taking her temperature, pulse and respiration, checking CRT and colour of her mucous membranes every five minutes and then every ten minutes once her body temperature had risen to 38°C.

7. Outcome of first aid emergency treatment:

Mable made a full recovery. Once her body temperature began to rise her other vital signs began to return to normal. We kept Mable in overnight to continue to monitor her progress and she was sent home the next day.

8. Dates to include: date of incident and full timescale range, if appropriate   15th March 04

Students comments, to include confirmation of your role in the procedures and any additional detail not given previously:

Comments:

I was confident in setting up the fluids for this dog as I have helped administer fluid therapy on previous occasions. It was important to remain calm for the owner who was very upset and needed reassurance. It was interesting monitoring her vital signs and this was a rewarding case to nurse.

The evidence in this log sheet is a true account of the case/procedures described and my involvement therein. The work undertaken in compiling the log is my own.

Student Veterinary Nurse's signature ....

Assessor's Comments:

The procedures and details recorded within this log sheet have been observed by ~~myself~~/a witness* (witness name A Vet ....) and have been carried out correctly and competently. *Please delete

Comments:

Having already established with the vet that Anne correctly prepared the necessary equipment for this case, we discussed the causes for raised and decreased vital signs. Anne has a good understanding of these and was able to correctly identify conditions that would result in abnormalities.

Assessor's name: ....

Assessor's signature: ....

Date: ....

Assessor's qualifications: ....

Case log 3.10 Log sheet 7A – Medical Nursing

Student veterinary nurse's name:		A Student		VN enrolment no:	E2004
1. Case details:	Species:	Feline		Age:	11 yr 6 mths
	Breed:	Domestic short haired (DSH)		Weight:	3.8 kg
				Sex:	Male entire

2. Case no. identification: Oliver

Assessor's comments:

3. Major presenting problems and history:

Dyspnoea – difficulty breathing in and out

4. Principle clinical findings:

On examination and auscultation of Oliver's chest, the vet identified mixed dyspnoea and a weak and irregular heart rate. He was also concerned that there may be fluid in the thorax.

5. Diagnostic procedures and tests: (a) State procedures and test(s) carried out in order to assist in the diagnosis of the condition. (b) Describe your involvement with these procedures.

Radiographs of the thorax – please refer to Case log 8a Oliver

Thoracocentesis – please refer to Case log 6a Oliver

Electrocardiogram (ECG) – the recording was sent away for a specialist to read – at the time of writing this case log, the results were not available.

6. Comment on clinical findings, test results and veterinary surgeon's diagnosis:

Please refer to Case logs 8a Rad 5 and 6a Lab 3/Oliver for the results and diagnosis.
It was important to keep Oliver calm throughout all the procedures so as not to stress him further and make his condition worse.

7. Medical treatment and Nursing, to include: *Medication and other treatments prescribed. Dietary management, Monitoring of progress and response to treatments. *Fluid therapy*
(details can be expanded in log sheet 7b.)

I initially gave Oliver oxygen via a face mask to help with his breathing. After the radiographs and thoracocentesis, he was hospitalized overnight.
On admission he was given 0.38 ml of Synulox (amoxicillin/clavulanate) a long-acting antibiotic and 0.5 ml Lasix furosemide (frusemide) a diuretic, both by subcutaneous injection.
I offered Oliver 100ml of fresh water – the amount was measured so that we could monitor how much he was drinking. He was also given sardines to try and encourage him to eat.
Oliver was then prescribed a 7-day course of furosemide (frusemide) tablets at an oral dose rate of ¼ tablet twice daily and an 8-day course of Fortekor (benazepril hydrochloride) at an oral dose rate of ½ tablet once a day.

8. Case summary and evaluation: e.g. the outcome, your role in case, information given to clients

While Oliver was in for 24 hours I played a large role as I was involved with the thoracocentesis, radiographs, ECG and monitoring him after treatment.
The vet gave the owners a guarded prognosis and advised further tests and treatment. As he is an elderly cat, Oliver's owners took him home to think about it. In view of the laboratory results which followed, the vet decided that neoplasia was more likely than a cardiac cause but

What factors did you consider when choosing a suitable kennel for Oliver?
A. One that was reasonably quiet away from dogs but in a position that made him easy to observe at all times.

How else might oxygen be administered to a conscious animal?
A. Via an oxygen tent using cling film over a buster collar or by enclosing the whole kennel with cling film and placing an open-ended supply of oxygen into the kennel.

continued overpage

Case log 3.10 – continued

decided to continue with frusemide and benazepril as no specific treatment/surgery would have been feasible in this case.

Date(s) to include: full timescale range, if appropriate ......
6 February to 7 February 05 ...... lab results 10 February ...

Student's comments and signature:

Comments

I found this a very interesting case as it involved several procedures being carried out and this was the first thoracocentesis I had seen.

The evidence in this log sheet is a true account of the case/procedures described and of my involvement therein. The work undertaken in compiling the log is my own.

Student veterinary nurse's signature ....

Assessor's statement:

The procedures and details recorded within this log sheet have been observed by myself/a witness* (witness's name ....)
and have been carried out correctly and competently. *Please delete

Comments:

Anne competently assisted with all the procedures and monitored Oliver during his hospitalization. Anne relayed information to Oliver's owners correctly and sympathetically.

Assessor's signature: ....   Assessor's name: ....

Assessor's qualifications: ....   Date: ....

Case log 3.11 Log sheet 8A – Radiography

Student veterinary nurse's name:		A Student		VN enrolment no:	E2004	
1. Case details:	Species:	Feline		Age:	11yr 6mths	
	Breed:	DSH		Weight:	3.8 kg	Sex: Male Entire
2. Case no. identification:		Rad 5	Date image produced	6 February 05		Assessor's comments:

3. Area to be radiographed and reason:

Thorax – Oliver has dyspnoea (difficulty breathing) and the vet suspects he may have fluid on his chest.

4. Patient preparation, to include: means of restraint e.g. manual, chemical (state medication used)

The vet decided not to give a premedicant as Oliver is dyspnoeic but it was also felt it would cause him more stress to try and restrain him while conscious and therefore 2 ml of Rapinovet (propofol) was administered intravenously.

When is it acceptable to hold animals manually for radiography?

A. Only in emergency situations where the animal may die as a result of giving a sedative or anaesthetic.

5. Recording equipment:	Screen type:	High-detail intensifying screen		Film type:	Slow film – high detail	Grid:	No
6. Exposure factors:	FFD:	75cm		KV:	60	MAs:	0.1

7. View e.g. ventrodorsal: *Dorsoventral*

8. Positioning of animal, to include: positioning aids used:

I placed Oliver on his sternum in the dorsoventral position. Sandbags were placed either side of his abdomen and his head and neck were placed in a natural position. His fore limbs were extended cranially and abducted. His hind legs were flexed in a frog position with sandbags placed over them.

Define the term abducted.

A. Pulled away from the body

continued overpage

Case log 3.11 – continued

I placed a marker on the cassette to indicate the right side of the thorax and a label was used stating Oliver's surname, the date and the X-ray number. Care was taken that both labels were within the primary beam but not obstructing the thorax.

9. Centring details (state anatomical landmarks):

I centred the primary beam on the fifth thoracic rib interspace just caudal to the body of the scapulae.

10. Collimation of primary beam (state anatomical landmarks):

I collimated to include both lateral skin surfaces and cranially to C7 and caudally to T13/L1 to include the thoracic inlet and the diaphragm.

11. Appraisal of radiographical quality to include:
Comments/action taken: ✔ = Satisfactory   X = unsatisfactory

| Positioning | ✔ | Collimation | ✔ | Centring | ✔ |
| Labelling | ✔ | Contrast | ✔ | Density | ✔ |

Comments and action taken if required:

Positioning, collimation and centring were good and the labels within the primary beam without obscuring any areas of interest. The contrast was satisfactory.

If artefacts were present, please state likely cause: *No artefacts were present.*

| Please indicate how the radiograph was processed: (Please tick box) | Manually ☐ | OR | Automatically ✔ |

12. Veterinary surgeon's diagnosis:

An accumulation of fluid was clearly visible on the radiographs and was likely to be causing Oliver's dyspnoea. The vet decided to perform thoracocentesis to drain Oliver's chest to relieve the clinical signs i.e. difficulty in breathing.

Why was Oliver not placed in lateral recumbency?
A. This would have improved his breathing

If artefacts were present on the developed radiograph, what action would you take?
A. Check with the vet if they required another x-ray to be taken. Try and establish whether the artefact was present before the film was developed or occurred during the developing process. Check the intensifying screens within the cassette and clean if necessary.

Student's comments and signature:

Comments:

The pleural cavity normally contains only sufficient fluid for adequate lubrication of the intrathoracic organs and the cavity lining and the excess fluid in this case was causing the dyspnoea.

The evidence in this log sheet is a true account of the case/procedure described and my involvement therein. The work undertaken in compiling the log is my own.

Student VN's signature ....

Assessor's statement:

The procedures and details recorded within this log sheet have been observed by myself/~~a witness~~* (witness's name ....) and have been carried out correctly and competently. *Please delete

Comments:

Anne and I have discussed the advantages and disadvantages of giving medication to a dyspnoeic patient. Her anatomical knowledge is good and positioning of patients together with collimation has improved. Anne always adheres to health and safety regulations.

Assessor's signature: ....

Assessor's qualifications: ....

Assessor's name: ....

Date: ....

Case log 3.12 Log sheet 6A – Laboratory and Diagnostic Aids

Student veterinary nurse's name:		*A Student*	VN enrolment no:	*E2004*
1. Case details:	Species:	*Feline*	Age:	*11yr 6mths*
	Breed:	*Domestic short haired (DSH)*	Weight:	*3.8 kg*
			Sex:	*Male entire*

2. Case no. identification: *LAB 3*

3. Type of procedure and reason for test:

Thoracocentesis – thora (thorax) co centesis (withdraw)
Oliver was diagnosed as having fluid on his chest and was dyspnoeic. Fluid was drained to relieve his clinical symptoms.

4. Preparation of animal and pretest procedures:

Oliver was still under very mild anaesthesia from the propofol given to enable radiographs to be taken of his chest.
Food or water would not have had to have been withdrawn for this procedure to have been undertaken other than for anaesthetic purposes.

5. Equipment and supplies required:

Electric clippers – cleaned and sprayed with Clippercide
Hibiscrub and cotton wool (1:20 dilution in warm water)
Surgical spirit
Sterile syringe
Sterile needle 23 g

Assessor's comments:

Can this procedure be carried out on a conscious patient?
A. Yes although a sedative is usually given.

What alternative to a needle could be used?
A. An over-the-needle catheter of a similar gauge.

Case log 3.12 – continued

Three-way tap
Surgical gloves
Ethylene diamine tetra-acetic acid (EDTA) tube
Plain tube

6. Preparation of equipment:

I cleaned the clippers using a toothbrush and then sprayed with Clippercide.
I laid all the remaining equipment out on a disposable drape and opened and handed to the vet in an aseptic manner.

7. Collection of sample:

I cleaned Oliver's chest in an aseptic manner. The vet wore surgical gloves and inserted the needle into the thoracic cavity and, using the connected syringe, withdrew fluid. A three-way tap was used to prevent air entering the chest when the syringe was removed for the fluid to be placed into the collecting tubes. A total of 120 ml was removed.
On placing the needle, the vet explained to me that the needle entered the thoracic cavity at a different intercostal space to that underlying the site of skin insertion. This is to help prevent air moving into the thorax when the needle is removed.

Date(s) sample collected and test carried out: ... 6 February 05 ....

Why is it necessary to carry this procedure out aseptically?
A. To prevent infection being introduced to the thorax and to prevent contamination of the sample being collected.

8. Preparation of sample for testing/storage and preservation, prior to dispatch:

The fluid was immediately placed into both an EDTA and plain tube which were labelled with the date, and the name of animal and owner.

9. Procedure(s) for test OR packaging and postage – method of dispatch (see guidance notes):

I ensured that the lids were securely on the tubes and then wrapped them in cotton wool.
I then placed the tubes into a small plastic bag and sealed it.

continued overpage

Case log 3.12 – continued

Having completed the appropriate laboratory request form, I placed this in a separate small plastic bag.

Both plastic bags were then placed into a jiffy bag, which I labelled with:
The full name and address of the external laboratory
The full name and address of our practice
Handle With Care – Veterinary Pathological Specimen.
I recorded the sample details in our laboratory file.
I posted the package in accordance with current Royal Mail guidelines.

I observed Anne correctly packaging the sample

10. Results of test:	Fluid was modified transudate and contained cell types highly suspicious of a neoplastic nature. On the basis of these results, a tentative diagnosis of lymphoma was made and the prognosis was very poor.

11. Normal ranges:	The pleural cavity normally contains only sufficient fluid for adequate lubrication of the intrathoracic organs and the cavity lining.

12. Examples of conditions which may give rise to abnormal ranges:

Q. When may air be present in the thorax?
A. Following trauma to the chest if a rib punctured a lung.

Pyothorax – an accumulation of pus in the thorax
Pneumothorax – an accumulation of air in the thorax
Foreign body – carcinoma

13. Possible reasons for inaccurate results:

Contamination of the sample – not collecting the sample aseptically, or placing the sample in a non-sterile tube.

Student VN's comments and signature:

Comments:

I enjoyed nursing Oliver and being involved with all the procedures as this made the nursing care more relevant and personal. Being an elderly cat made the diagnosis easier for me to accept and, although little can be done for Oliver in the long term, the medication should make him more comfortable and improve his current quality of life.

The evidence in this log sheet is a true account of the case/procedures described and my involvement therein. The work undertaken in compiling the log is my own.

Student veterinary nurse's signature: ....

Assessor's statement:

The procedures and details recorded within this log sheet have been observed by myself/~~a witness~~* (witness's name.............................)
and have been carried out correctly and competently. *Please delete

Comments:

Anne efficiently collected and prepared the equipment needed for collecting the sample itself and for posting it afterwards. She observed the relevant health and safety protocols.

Assessor's signature: ....   Assessor's name: ....

Assessor's qualifications: ....   Date: ....

Case log 3.13 Log sheet 7B – Fluid Management

Student veterinary nurse's name:	A Student		VN enrolment no.:	E2004	
1. Case details:	Breed:	Golden Retriever	Age:	10yr 8mths	
	Species:	Canine	Weight:	16 kg	Sex:
					Female Neutered
2. Case no. identification:	Bramble		Assessor's comments:		

3. Reason for administering fluid:

The veterinary surgeon in charge of this case decided for Bramble to be administered with intravenous fluid therapy in an attempt to correct her circulatory collapse caused by her shocked state.

4. Type of fluid selected: *According to veterinary surgeon's instructions.*

The vet chose Haemaccel. This type of fluid is known as a colloid. There are two types of colloid:
plasma volume replacers e.g. dextrans
plasma volume expanders e.g. Haemaccel.

5. Reason for choice of fluid and route of administration:

The vet considered this type of fluid to be the most suitable as he evaluated Bramble to be in circulatory collapse as a result of shock. Her circulation was compromised with her heart being unable to sustain sufficient output to the peripheral tissues with blood being shifted to her vital organs, e.g. the heart, lungs and brain.

6. Equipment and supplies: *State what was selected and how it was prepared in order to administer the fluids.*

One × Haemaccel 500 ml
One giving set
One skin cleanser swab soaked in dilute Hibiscrub
One surgical spirit swab
Micropore tape
One 20 gauge × 1.25 inch catheter
Bandaging material: Soffban, Vetwrap.

continued overpage

Setting up the fluid bag and giving set:

(1) The expiry date on the fluids was checked. (2) Fluids were warmed to body temperature. (3) The outer package concealing the fluids was removed. (4) The seal to the giving port was broken. (5) The giving set bag was opened and the giving set regulator was closed. (6) The giving set was inserted into the fluid bag without contaminating any of the set. (7) The drip chamber was squeezed until the drip chamber became half full with fluid. (8) The giving set regulator was opened to allow the fluid to fill up the giving set tubing and run through to ensure no air bubbles were present within the tubing.

Selecting a suitable vein and gauge catheter:

(1) One of Bramble's cephalic veins situated in the fore limb was chosen in order for the fluids to be administered intravenously: (2) The site over the vein was clipped with electric clippers. (3) A skin preparation of chlorhexidine was used to cleanse the skin thoroughly. (4) Surgical spirit was used to wipe over the site. The catheter was inserted into the cephalic vein and secured in place using Micropore tape. (5) The giving line was attached to the catheter and secured with Micropore. (7) The catheter was flushed with heparinized saline. (8) A bandage was applied over the catheter and giving line.

7. Fluid therapy plan: (a) Estimated total fluid deficit. (b) Rate of administration (include ml per hour and drip rate) Show how volume (a) and rates (b) were calculated.

No estimated fluid deficit was calculated in this case

Maintenance fluid rate – 50 ml/kg/24 hours

50 ml × 16 kg × 1 day = 800 ml/24 hours
800 ml ÷ 24 hours = 33 ml/hour
33 ml ÷ 60 = 0.55 ml/minute
0.55 ml ÷ 60 = 0.009 ml/second
0.009 ml × 20 (drops/ml – giving set) = 0.18 (rounded up to 0.2) drops/second = 1 drop every 5 seconds

Bramble received approximately 250 ml of the intended infusion before she died.

8. Summary of fluid therapy plan: any revisions to the initial plan

The initial fluid therapy plan was not completed owing to Bramble dying during treatment.

Case log 3.13 – continued

9. Monitoring of the animal: (a) Monitoring of administration, urine output, vital signs, etc. and animal's progress. (b) A recording chart/record used by you to monitor this animal must be attached

The following monitoring was carried out on Bramble while the Haemaccel was being administered:
Pulse including rate and rhythm
Mucous membrane colour
Capillary refill time
Respiratory rate
Mean arterial blood pressure
Body temperature
Urine output
Skin turgor.

Date(s), to include: full timescale range, if appropriate 10.02.04

State the clinical signs of shock
A. Weak, rapid pulse
Increased heart rate (tachycardia)
Pale, clammy mucous membranes
Increased capillary refill time
Shallow, rapid respirations
Hypothermia, cold extremities
Muscle weakness
Depressed level of consciousness
Reduced renal output.

How often were these checks carried out?
A. Every 5 minutes.

Student's comments and signature:

Comments:

Bramble's death was not unexpected as the vet gave a guarded prognosis when he admitted her. I am confident in assembling fluids and monitoring patients and in Bramble's case her vital signs were affected by her being clinically in shock.

The evidence in this log sheet is a true account of the case/procedures described and of my involvement therein. The work undertaken in compiling the log is my own.

Student veterinary nurse's signature ....

Assessor's statement:

The procedures and details recorded within this log sheet have been observed by myself/~~a witness~~* (witness's name ....) and have been carried out correctly and competently. *Please delete

Comments:

Anne confidently prepared and assembled the equipment. Her understanding of shock and physiology are excellent. She monitored Bramble professionally.

Assessor's signature: .... Assessor's name: ....

Assessor's qualifications: .... Date: ....

Case log 3.14 Log sheet 7B – Fluid Management

Student veterinary nurse's name:		A Student	VN enrolment no:	E2004
1. Case details:	Breed:	Golden retriever	Age:	10yr 8mths
	Species:	Canine	Weight:	16 kg
			Sex:	F Neutered
2. Case no. identification:		Bramble		

3. Reason for administering fluid:

In an attempt to correct circulatory collapse caused by shock.

4. Type of fluid selected: According to veterinary surgeon's instructions.

Haemaccel – plasma volume expander.

5. Reason for choice of fluid and route of administration:

To boost circulation as in a shocked patient circulation is compromised.

6. Equipment and supplies: *State what was selected and how it was prepared in order to administer the fluids.*

One × Haemaccel 500 ml – checked date of expiry and warmed to body temperature approximately 38°C
One giving set – packaging checked for sterility
One skin cleanser swab soaked in dilute Hibiscrub (chlorhexidine)
One surgical spirit swab
Micropore tape
On 20 gauge × 1.25 inch catheter
Bandaging material: Soffban, Vetwrap
Having first washed my hands I then:
● removed the outer packaging from drip and giving set
● broke the seal to the giving port

Assessor's Comments:

We discussed this in more detail and Anne was able to explain that in animals suffering from shock, blood is sent to vital organs e.g. heart, lungs and brain and away from the peripheral tissues.

continued overpage

Case log 3.14 – continued

- closed the giving set regulator
- inserted the giving set into the fluid bag without contaminating any of the set
- filled the drip chamber by squeezing it until half full with fluid
- opened the giving set regulator and run through the fluids slowly to ensure no air bubbles were present within the tubing.

7. Fluid therapy plan: (a) Estimated total fluid deficit. (b) Rate of administration (include ml per hour and drip rate). *Show how volume (a) and rates (b) were calculated.*

No estimated fluid deficit was calculated in this case.

Maintenance fluid rate – 50 ml/kg/24 h

50 ml × 16 kg × 1 day = 800 ml/24 h
800 ml ÷ 24 h = 33 ml/h
33 ml ÷ 60 = 0.55 ml/min
0.55 ml ÷ 60 = 0.009 ml/s
0.009 ml × 20 (drops/ml – giving set) = 0.18 (rounded up to 0.2) drops/second = 1 drop every 5 seconds.

Bramble received approximately 250 ml of the intended infusion before she died.

8. Summary of fluid therapy plan (any revisions to the initial plan):

The initial fluid therapy plan was not completed owing to Bramble dying during treatment.

9. Monitoring of the animal: (a) Monitoring of administration, urine output, vital signs, etc. and animal's progress. (b) A recording chart/record used by you to monitor this animal must be attached.

I carried out the following monitoring on Bramble every 5 minutes while the Haemaccel was being administered:
 Pulse including rate and rhythm
 Mucous membrane colour
 Capillary refill time
 Respiratory rate

State the clinical signs of shock
A. Weak, rapid pulse
Increased heart rate (tachycardia)
Pale, clammy mucous membranes
Increased capillary refill time
Shallow, rapid respirations
Hypothermia, cold extremities
Muscle weakness
Depressed level of consciousness
Reduced renal output

Mean arterial blood pressure
Body temperature
Urine output
Skin turgor.

Date(s), to include: full timescale range, if appropriate 10.02.04

Student's comments and signature:

Comments:

Bramble's death was not unexpected as the vet gave a guarded prognosis when he admitted her. I am confident in assembling fluids and monitoring patients and in Bramble's case her vital signs were affected by her being clinically in shock.

The evidence in this log sheet is a true account of the case/procedures described and of my involvement therein. The work undertaken in compiling the log is my own.

Student veterinary nurse's signature ....

Assessor's statement:

The procedures and details recorded within this log sheet have been observed by myself/~~a witness~~* (witness's name ....)
and have been carried out correctly and competently. *Please delete

Comments:

Anne confidently prepared and assembled the equipment. Her understanding of shock and physiology are excellent. She monitored Bramble professionally.

Assessor's signature: ....   Assessor's name: ....

Assessor's qualifications: ....   Date: ....

Case log 3.15 Log sheet 5A – Basic Equine Management

Student veterinary nurse's name:		A Student	VN enrolment no.:	E2004
1. Case details:	Species:	Equine	Age:	8 years
	Breed:	Warmblood Brood Mare	Weight:	525 kg
				Sex: Mare

2. Case no. identification: Bubbles

3. Reason for hospitalization:

Retrobulbar mass to the left eye with a yellow mucopurulent discharge.
Non-odourous mucopurulent discharge from left nostril.
Pyrexic – temperature was 39.4°C.
Mare due to foal in 30 days.

Assessor's comments:

How many days gestation is Bubbles?
A. 310 days

4. Type of accommodation and bedding material used, to include (any relevant environmental factors)

Internal loose box. The mare was stabled in a large hospital box measuring 5 × 4 m (16 by 12 feet) as she is heavily in foal.
A deep bed of barley straw was provided.
A heat lamp was available to provide extra warmth if required.

Why was straw the bedding of choice?
A. Woodshavings are not suitable for new born foals as they can block their nostrils.

5. Accommodation cleaning protocol, to include: type of disinfectant and dilution, mechanical cleaning procedures, frequency of cleaning and disposal of waste:

I mucked out the stable twice daily. Faeces and urine soaked bedding was removed and new straw was put down.
   In between patients, the boxes are disinfected with Trigene diluted 1:200. The walls and floors are scrubbed and washed with warm water and dilute Trigene and left to dry naturally.

6. Feeding Regimen:

The mare is normally kept on grass at home. Her diet had been supplemented at home with hard feed and hay in preparation for foaling. While stabled at the clinic I monitored her carefully as a change in diet may cause colonic impaction.

- *Soaked hay was offered ad lib.*
- *A small quantity of bran mash was given twice daily.*
- *Both hay and hard feed were fed from the floor to help the sinus drain under gravity.*
- *Water was provided ad lib.*

How long was the hay soaked for?
A. 20 minutes and then allowed to drain.

7. Nursing care and monitoring of the animal: please give details of grooming, wound management, foot care, cleaning, monitoring of vital signs and 'TLC'.

I carried out the following:
- *Temperature, pulse and respiratory rates were monitored twice daily and recorded.*
- *Groomed daily – body, mane and tail brushed using a body brush (see student comments).*
- *All feet picked out.*
- *Nostrils and eyes wiped clean with gauze swabs soaked in warm water.*
- *The frontal and maxillary sinuses were trephined to aid treatment – daily flushing with 4 litres of water was therefore required.*
- *The lower trephine hole was cleaned with swabs and dilute povidine–iodine solution and then re-plugged with a gauze swab after each flushing to prevent the hole from healing over.*
- *To aid drainage from the sinuses the mare was walked daily in the fresh air and hand grazed.*

Date(s) specify duration of hospitalization 30.03.04 to 06.04.04 (7 days).

What dilution of povidine–iodine can be used on eyes and mucous membranes?
A. 0.1–0.2%

Describe how the sinuses were flushed.
A. Water was pumped into the sinus via the indwelling Foley catheter using a garden spray pump.

8. Medication administered: (details can be cross-referenced to Log 5c)

Benzyl penicillin (Crystapen) 10 Mega 6 g, Gentamicin (Pangram) 4 g and Eltenac (Telzenac) 350 mg were given intravenously
Phenylbutazone (Equipalzone) 2 g was given intravenously
Betamethasone (Betsolan) drops were applied to the prolapsed conjunctiva four times daily
Metronidazole (Metronex paste) 10 g was given twice daily by mouth to reduce bacterial load within the sinus.

continued overpage

Case log 3.15 – continued

Student's comments, to include: the part the student has played in this case:

Comments:

Whether to groom a patient will depend upon the degree of illness for which it is being treated. Most horses benefit from contact in the form of hand rubbing or grooming with a selection of brushes. The veterinary surgeon must always be consulted before grooming and care must be taken of any drains, lavage systems, etc. Always groom gently and keep the horse out of draughts. If wearing a rug, do not strip completely; rather 'quarter' the horse.

I was the nurse responsible for the day-to-day care of this patient. I assisted with the trephining procedure by preparing the site aseptically and also helping with the flushing of the sinuses.

Copy of hospitalization record attached   YES ☐   NO ✔

The evidence in this log sheet is a true account of the case/procedures described and my involvement therein. The work undertaken in compiling the log is my own.

Student veterinary nurse's signature ....

Assessor's statement:

The procedures and details recorded within this log sheet have been observed by myself/~~a witness~~* (witness's name..)
and have been carried out correctly and competently. *Please delete

Comments:

Amy demonstrated a good understanding of the anatomy associated with this condition. She nursed the patient well and followed all instructions regarding the aftercare, feeding, grooming, etc.

Assessor's signature: ....   Assessor's name: ....

Assessor's qualifications: ....   Date: ....

Case log 3.16 Log sheet 7A – Medical Nursing

Student veterinary nurse's name:		A Student	VN enrolment no:	E2004
1. Case details:	Species:	Equine	Age:	5 years
	Breed:	Thoroughbred	Weight:	400 kg
			Sex:	Mare
2. Case no. identification:		Dolce		

3. Major presenting problems and history:

The mare presented with signs of respiratory distress, weight loss and inappetence and had been ill for 4 months.
She had responded to previous systemic antibiotics but symptoms returned once each course had finished.

4. Principle clinical findings:

- *Dyspnoeic*
- *Tachypnoeic*
- *Pyrexic – rectal temperature 40°C. For normal temperature ranges, see Appendix 4.*

5. Diagnostic procedures and tests: (a) State procedures and test(s) carried out in order to assist in the diagnosis of the condition. (b) Describe your involvement with these procedures.

- *Standing thoracic radiography*
- *Diagnostic ultrasonography*
- *Thoracocentesis and cytology*

6. Comment on clinical findings, test results and veterinary surgeon's diagnosis:

- *Thoracic auscultation revealed an absence of lung sounds ventrally on both sides.*
- *Cardiac sounds were audible widely and bilaterally.*
- *Thoracic percussion did not provoke a pain response; however, there was reduced resonance.*

Assessor's comments:

What part did you play in respect of the diagnostic tests?
A. I developed the radiographs, and held Dolce for the ultrasonography.

continued overpage

Case log 3.16 – *continued*

These findings were suggestive of pleural effusion.

- Radiographs confirmed the presence of a pleural effusion.
- Ultrasonography revealed a bilateral, homogenous hypoechoic pleural effusion.
- Thoracocentesis revealed an exudative effusion; 10 litres of yellow turbid fluid were drained.
- Bacteriological culture of the fluid yielded a profuse growth of beta-haemolytic Streptococcus sp. Chronic pleuropneumonia was diagnosed.

7. Medical treatment and nursing, to include: Medication and other treatments prescribed. Dietary management. Monitoring of progress and response to treatments. *Fluid therapy* *(details can be expanded in Log sheet 7b).*

- *An indwelling chest drain (28 French gauge) was placed aseptically in the right-hand side with a one-way valve and sutured in place. This was left open to drain continuously following the initial drainage (see above).*
- *I checked the site of the chest drain for signs of swelling and leakage.*
- *A long-stay central venous catheter was placed in the left jugular to aid administration of benzyl penicillin (Crystapen) 10 mg/kg i.v. twice daily, gentamicin (Genta 100) 6.6 mg/kg i.v. once daily and flunixin megluine (Finadyne) 0.25 mg/kg i.v. four times daily.*
- *Dolce was experiencing pain and was therefore reluctant to eat. It was important to tempt her to eat and keep her interested and bright. I offered bran mashes, pasture mix, carrots and apples.*

As she improved, her fibre intake was increased by offering 'Hifi' and good quality haylage. Grooming was carried out taking care of the indwelling catheter and chest drain.

8. Case summary and evaluation: e.g. the outcome, your role in case, information given to clients.

- Repeated thoracic ultrasonograpy after 24 hours showed a reduction of the effusion bilaterally.
- The horse's demeanour improved over the first few days of treatment.
- Her appetite increased and she appeared much brighter.
- After 9 days' hospitalization, the mare was discharged with the intravenous catheter still in place to allow administration of benzyl penicillin and gentamicin at home by the owner.
- Catheter care was discussed in detail with the owner.

Date(s) to include: full timescale range, if appropriate 9 days from 24 January 2004 to 1 February 2004

Student's comments and signature:

Comments:

Catheter care was extremely important as the mare needed long-term antibiotic therapy. Diagnostic ultrasonography was very useful in this case, both for aiding the initial diagnosis and for monitoring the progression of the disease and the response to treatment.

The evidence in this log sheet is a true account of the case/procedures described and of my involvement therein. The work undertaken in compiling the log is my own.

Student veterinary nurse's signature ....

Assessor's statement:

The procedures and details recorded within this log sheet have been observed by myself/a witness* (witness's name ....) and have been carried out correctly and competently. *Please delete as appropriate

Comments:

Amy was responsible for the care of this mare's chest drain and took the major responsibility for her care. She demonstrated excellent nursing skills throughout.

Assessor's signature: .... Assessor's name: ....

Assessor's qualifications: .... Date: ....

Figure 3.8 Appendix 4 Normal vital signs.

Foal newborn	
Pulse rate (b/min)	100–128
Respiration rate (/min)	14–15
Rectal temperature (°C)	38.5–39.5
Capillary refill time (s)	<2
Foal (7 days)	
Pulse rate (b/min)	80–20
Respiration rate (/min)	14–16
Rectal temperature (°C)	38.0–39.0
Capillary refill time (s)	<2
Foal (3 months)	
Pulse rate (b/min)	60–100
Respiration rate (/min)	14–15
Rectal temperature (°C)	37.5–38.0
Capillary refill time (s)	<2
Pony	
Pulse rate (b/min)	45–55
Respiration rate (/min)	12–15
Rectal temperature (°C)	37.5–38.0
Capillary refill time (s)	<2
Thoroughbred	
Pulse rate (b/min)	35–45
Respiration rate (/min)	12–15
Rectal temperature (°C)	37.5–38.0
Capillary refill time (s)	<2
Thoroughbred (fit)	
Pulse rate (b/min)	25–40
Respiration rate (/min)	10–5
Rectal temperature (°C)	37.5–38.5
Capillary refill time (s)	<2

A Student 10 April 04
The Assessor MRCVS 17 April 04

Welsh Pony Filly Dido
- 9c Preparation and assisting surgical procedures (Case log 3.17)
- Surgical instrument appendices 5 and 6 (Figs 3.9, 3.10).

Thoroughbred Lillymay
- 9c Preparation and assisting surgical procedures (Case log 3.18).

Case log 3.17 Log sheet 9C – Preparation and Assisting Surgical Procedures

Student veterinary nurse's name:		*A Student*	VN enrolment no:	*E2004*
1. Case details:	Species:	*Equine*	Age:	*8 weeks*
	Breed:	*Welsh Pony*	Weight:	*100 kg*
			Sex:	*Filly*

2. Case no. identification: *Dido*

	Assessor's comments:

3. Surgical procedure:

Repair of ruptured corneal ulcer

Which eye?
A. Right eye

4. Preparation of instruments, surgical equipment and materials:

General routine surgical kit, see Appendix 5, plus ophthalmic instruments, see Appendix 6.

5. Preparation of the animal for surgery:

- *A long-stay Mila catheter was inserted aseptically into the left jugular vein.*
- *100 mg flunixin meglumine (Finadyne) was given preoperatively by intravenous (i.v.) injection.*
- *I applied Atropine drops (atropine sulphate drops 1%) and gentamicin drops (Genticin eye drops 0.3%) topically to the right eye.*
- *Romifidine (Sedivet) 100 mg was administered i.v. 5 minutes prior to induction with Ketamine (Narkatan) 250 mg i.v. plus 5 mg diazepam i.v.*
- *Anaesthesia was maintained with halothane in oxygen.*
- *Following induction, the foal was intubated using a size 16 silicone cuffed endotracheal tube.*
- *I clipped the eyelids and periorbital region and aseptically prepared the area. The eye was lavaged with sterile saline 0.9%.*

What other eye preparation was undertaken?
A. K–Y Jelly was applied prior to clipping to prevent hair from being introduced into the eye.

continued overpage

Case log 3.17 – continued

- *Rectal gloves were placed over the feet and distal limit to minimize contamination of the theatre.*
- *The foal was then hobbled and transported into theatre. Care was taken to ensure the foal was positioned correctly to avoid potential damage to the back muscles and vasculature.*

6. Assisting during the surgical procedure:

The foal was placed in left lateral recumbency and maintained on isoflurane in oxygen.
I assisted the veterinary surgeon to put on a sterile surgical disposable gown and gloves.
I opened the disposable drapes and passed these to the vet.
These were used to prevent contamination of the surgical site by hair and the immediate environment.
I opened surgical instruments as required and passed them aseptically to the surgeon.

What are the advantages of using paper-based disposable gowns and drapes?
A. They are water-repellent and labour saving as they are pre-sterilized.

7. Recovery from surgery (postoperative care):

I assisted with the following:
On completion of surgery the eye was lavaged with sterile 0.9% saline solution and gentamicin drops were applied to the eye.
A urinary catheter was passed to evacuate the bladder.
The foal was returned to the recovery box and placed in right lateral recumbency.
She was given 2 mg xylazine (Virbaxyl) i.v.
She was extubated 10 minutes later and oxygen was administered via a nasopharyngeal tube.
She made an uneventful and smooth recovery and was standing 30 minutes after being placed in the recovery box.
She returned to her stable an hour later and was placed with her mother to reduce stress.
The foal was closely observed to ensure she was drinking normally.

Date(s) to include full timescale range if appropriate. 15.07.04 to 25.07.04 (5 days)

Case log 3.17 – continued

Student's comments and signature:

Comments:

I was involved with the care of the foal during the surgical procedure and during its stay at the hospital. It was a particularly difficult case as the foal was kept with the dam and both were not well handled.

The evidence in this log sheet is a true account of the case/procedures described and of my involvement therein. The work undertaken in compiling the log is my own.

Student veterinary nurse's signature:..

Assessor's statement:

The procedures and details recorded within this log sheet have been observed by myself/a witness* (witness's name ....) and have been carried out correctly and competently. *Please delete

Comments:

Despite being a nursing challenge, Amy demonstrated excellent handling and nursing skills both within the theatre and during the postoperative care.

Assessor's signature: ....   Assessor's name: ....

Assessor's qualifications: ....   Date: ....

Case log 3.18 Log sheet 9C – Preparation and Assisting Surgical Procedures

Student veterinary nurse's name:		A Student	VN enrolment no.:		E2004
1. Case details:	Species:	Equine	Age:	12 years	
	Breed:	Thoroughbred	Weight:	450 kg	
			Sex:		Mare

2. Case no. identification:

Lillymay

3. Surgical procedure:

Removal of granulosa cell tumour of the right ovary.

4. Preparation of instruments, surgical equipment and materials:

See Appendix 5 plus:
TA 90 Stapler
Doyens bowel clamps.

5. Preparation of the animal for surgery:

The patient was starved for 36 hours prior to surgery to allow the majority of the gastrointestinal tract to be emptied.
Shoes were removed.
I groomed her thoroughly to prevent environmental contamination of the theatre.
A jugular catheter was placed aseptically in the left jugular vein for venous access.
A premidicant of 25 mg acepromazine was given intramuscularly before entering the knockdown box.
I clipped the surgical site using size 40 blades approximately 30 cm to each side of the linea alba.
Loose hair was removed from the surgical site. Wearing gloves, I used a lint-free swab to wash the area using chlorhexidine (Hibiscrub). I began at the incision site and worked out towards the edge of the clipped area. The swab was then discarded and the process repeated using a clean swab until there was no discoloration on the white swab. The area was then sprayed with 70% alcohol solution to remove any remaining detergent.
Once anaesthetized, the patient was intubated and isoflurane in oxygen was administered via a circle circuit.

Assessor's comments:

Why are shoes removed for surgery?
A. To prevent damage to the patient and recovery box during induction and recovery

continued overpage

6. Assisting during the surgical procedure:

I carried out the skin preparation as described above.
I passed the surgical gown and gloves to the veterinary surgeon and assisted during the operation by passing the disposable drapes, surgical instruments and suture material when requested.

7. Recovery from surgery (postoperative care):

The Teflon catheter was removed and a Mila catheter inserted in the jugular vein.
During recovery the mare was catheterized to evacuate the bladder to promote a smooth recovery. If the bladder is full, the horse may try to stand before it is ready to do so.
The mare was box rested following surgery. I observed the surgical wound routinely for signs of swelling and exudates but, as she was very difficult to handle, I was unable to feel the wound for signs of heat. There was some oedema, which was to be expected postoperatively.
The mare was given a laxative diet and monitored for signs of impactions as she was not very mobile.
I walked her out for grass three times a day for 5 minutes to relieve the oedema and the risk of impactions.
I monitored her temperature, pulse and respiration twice daily.

Date(s) to include full timescale range if appropriate. 24.09.04 to 30.09.04 (7 days)

Why was the catheter changed?
A. A Mila catheter can be left in the vein for up to 21 days as it is made from a less thrombogenic polyurethane.

Student's comments and signature:

Comments:

This patient was very difficult to handle and her trust had to be gained before I was able to work safely around her.

The evidence in this log sheet is a true account of the case/procedures described and of my involvement therein. The work undertaken in compiling the log is my own.

Student veterinary nurse's signature:..

Assessor's statement:

The procedures and details recorded within this log sheet have been observed by myself/a witness* (witness's name ....)
and have been carried out correctly and competently. *Please delete

Comments:

Amy performed the nursing care very competently despite the temperament of the mare making her job very difficult.

Assessor's signature: .... Assessor's name: ....

Assessor's qualifications: .... Date: ....

Figure 3.9 Appendix 5 General equine surgical kit.

1 × Scalpel knife handle
1 × Mayo scissors straight 6.5 inch
1 × Mayo scissors straight 5.5 inch
1 × Metzenbaum scissors straight 7.25 inch
2 × Allis tissue forceps 4/5 teeth
4 × Backhaus towel holding forceps 3.5 inch
4 × Spencer Wells artery forceps straight 5 inch
4 × Spencer Wells artery forceps curved 5 inch
1 × Gillies combined scissors and needle holder
1 × Olsen Hegar needle holders
1 × Dissecting Bendover forceps
1 × Lanes forceps
10 × gauze swabs
1 × size 1 curved triangular cutting needle
1 × size 5 curved triangular cutting needle
1 × size 12 curved triangular cutting needle

A Student 26 July 04
The Assessor MRCVS 30 July 04

Figure 3.10 Appendix 6 Additional equine surgical instrument kit.

The following instruments are in addition to a general surgical kit:

Ophthalmic Surgery

Size 11 scalpel blade
Fine dissecting forceps
Fine scissors
Corneal scissors
Capsular forceps
Iris repository
Needle holders
Eyelid speculum
Irrigating cannula

A Student 26th July 04
The Assessor 30th July 04

SUPPORTING THE STUDENT

Mentoring

Depending on the number of students and assessors within a practice, it may be necessary to allocate students to specific assessors. The student:assessor ratio depends on the experience of the assessors, the time they have to carry out their role and the number and level of students within the practice. Ideally, the ratio should be about 1:3 if the assessor is qualified and experienced. Although it is expected that a named assessor will perform the majority of assessing along with the tutorials and reviews, all assessors are likely to work with all of the students at some point, especially if one assessor is off work for any reason. Also, specialist assessments may need to be performed by a member of staff who is more suitably qualified – for example, where one vet holds a certificate in radiography.

As an assessor you will act as tutor and advisor while the students study for their nursing NVQ. You will be responsible for observing the majority of their practical assessments, holding tutorial sessions with them and helping them plan and keep track of their progress. Having a good working relationship means that the students should refer any queries they may have to you. If there are other assessors in the practice, they can also be involved with assessing the students. It may be, for instance, that there is a member of staff who specializes in radiography or ultrasonography; it would therefore be ideal for them to act as evidence gatherer for some cases within the diagnostic imaging and radiography unit and module. What is not appropriate, however, is for individual assessors within a practice to be responsible for assessing only specific units. Rather, it is expected that all assessors will work with all of the students at some point during their nurse training. Where there is more than one assessor in a practice, 'in-house' meetings should be held to discuss the progress of students and to allocate future assessments to specific staff where relevant.

Tutorials

The aim of a good tutorial is to assist students to learn and build their confidence through confidential mentoring including:

- setting agreed targets and action plans
- educational and study support
- guidance in gathering evidence to meet Occupational Standards
- guidance on portfolio development and progression
- regular reviewing and checking of progress
- pastoral support
- support in the development of social and personal skills
- continual contact between the assessor, management team and student to ensure that they feel valued.

Each week some time needs to be spent with students on a one-to-one basis to give them feedback on their case logs and agree an action plan

Figure 3.11 Study time inventory.	
Day	**Hours**
Monday	
Tuesday	
Wednesday	
Thursday	
Friday	

for their next cases. The timing of tutorials is crucial to their success. These must be held frequently and be structured, but there must also be some flexibility to allow for impromptu meetings to deal with issues as they arise. All tutorial time must be recorded within the action plan or tutorial record.

The key components of an effective tutorial are:

- preparation
- setting targets
- listening
- keeping a record
- asking questions.

The practice is also expected to provide some theoretical input to support the day release college courses. Any time spent instructing a student, whether it is formally or over the operating table, should be recorded in the tutorial record.

Time management

Many of us have problems juggling time to meet all the priorities in life. It is not that we are lazy or bad time managers; it just seems that there is so much to do! To enable students to see how much study time they have, ask them to make a list of the time spent at college, work, travelling, eating, sleeping, etc. They should then make a quick inventory of the study time available during the week using a form like that in Figure 3.11. You can help them determine a schedule for the number of cases they should be writing up each week by referring to the portfolio tracking records and by working out the number of cases they have to complete.

CONTINUING PROFESSIONAL DEVELOPMENT FOR ASSESSORS

It is a mandatory requirement that all assessors remain occupationally competent and undertake continuing professional development (CPD) activities. These may involve attending veterinary or nursing congresses or a 1-day course, or undertaking further professional development and qualification. In addition, all assessors must attend at least one meeting per year held by their VNAC. The internal verifiers at the VNAC will have attended at least one meeting each per year held by the RCVS external verifiers and in this way are able to disseminate news, information regarding industry changes and awarding body requirements directly to their assessors. In addition, this is an excellent way to discuss ideas and problems with fellow assessors, particularly if you are a sole assessor within a practice. Copies of all certificates of attendance should be kept within the practice as evidence of CPD undertaken.

KEEPING ASSESSMENT DOCUMENTATION WITHIN THE TP

Producing and maintaining documentation is essential for providing evidence that assessment is taking place within a TP. However, it is possible to rationalize the amount of paperwork generated during the assessment process at the same time as ensuring that evidence of planning, tracking, feedback and review are maintained as described earlier in this chapter. The essential information that must be kept includes:

- *student details*; you may wish to have a confidential file for each student containing the following:
  - enrolment details
  - records of holiday and sickness during the training period
  - copies of all correspondence with or concerning the student
  - copies of individual module summary sheets identifying the types of evidence generated
  - tutorial records; the 'assessment planning and tutorial records' from the portfolio can be used and copies kept
  - all formal assessment documentation
  - college schemes of work and reports
  - notification of student change of employment or centre, where appropriate

- *assessor details*:
  - copy of original D32,33 or A1 certificate, which must be signed as having been authenticated
  - copies of CPD attendance certificates
  - IV assessor observation reports
  - IV reports and action taken on portfolio verification
  - minutes of assessor meetings, where there is more than one assessor in a TP

- *general details*:
  - memorandum of agreement
  - TP application form
  - IV reports – approval and monitoring
  - correspondence with VNAC and RCVS
  - minutes of staff meetings.

FREQUENTLY ASKED QUESTIONS AND ANSWERS

○ *Should case logs be typed or handwritten?*

● Both forms are acceptable. However, typed logs have the advantage of access to spell-check facilities, and medical spell-checks are also available. The completed case logs must follow the same format as those within the portfolio and great care must be taken when downloading them to ensure that all sections of each log sheet are included as in the originals and completed accordingly.

○ *When can students begin completing their portfolio case logs?*

● Portfolio case logs must be completed only during the period of enrolment, and the dates of treatment and assessor's signature must reflect this. Some theoretical input is recommended before starting some of the modules. Assessments are a means of identifying how much a student knows and is able to do and must therefore be undertaken only when students are ready and confident enough to produce evidence to demonstrate their competence. Although it is expected that the students demonstrate progression throughout a unit/module, first-time experiences are ideally not logged as students cannot be expected to be competent on the first occasion they undertake a task.

○ *Should a copy of the portfolio be kept?*

● Yes – imagine if a student lost the original. An actual photocopy would be the only way of having copies of the assessor's handwritten comments, signature or any questions. Case logs are better photocopied immediately they are assessed to reduce the time spent in bulk copying. An electronic copy will not suffice.

○ *What is the recommended timescale for assessing case logs once they are completed?*

● Assessment will involve the assessor(s) discussing the case log with individual students, asking questions and recording their answers, either in the margins of the actual case log or on a separate sheet, and then signing off the log itself. This should be done during the weekly tutorials; therefore the date of assessment will reflect this and should be within 2 weeks of the date of treatment.

○ *Can correction fluid be used to delete client details?*

● No, correction fluid should not be used in the portfolio. Confidential details should be obliterated by being crossed out in pen. Where an error is made, the student should neatly draw a line through it and write in the new details or information.

○ *How often should I hold tutorials?*

● Part of the 3 hours each student should receive each week, or 7 hours if not attending a college course, must be spent having a one-to-one tutorial with the assessor. Having regular tutorials enables you to discuss students' progress and sort out promptly any difficulties they encounter. During the remaining time, you will be observing your students during their normal working day, questioning them while working alongside them and possibly also holding 'teaching' sessions on specific topics. All of the above should be recorded within the assessment planning and tutorial record, which is currently annexe F of the portfolio.

○ Are appendices recommended?

● Yes. An appendix is a good base on which to build information within the portfolio. Each time a particular procedure arises, your students can then refer to the specific appendix number. However, make sure they do not omit relevant information to specific cases by merely referring to an appendix. An entry was once read about a gerbil that, according to the appendix, was housed in a dog kennel on a vet bed!

○ Are 'student comments' necessary in all the case logs?

● Yes. This box is for your students to make reflective comments about their roles and experiences during the nursing and monitoring care of individual patients. Such comments can provide a real insight into their personal development during their training. A nurse is expected to learn from the experience of actually doing the job and this involves reflection, questioning and self-criticism.

○ Should case logs be written in rough first?

● Your students may be prefer to write the first case log in each module in rough and discuss its contents with you; you will then be able to confirm whether or not they are on the right track. Thereafter, each case log should be written up and presented for assessment as a final copy. You may then ask your students questions about the content of individual case logs, terminology used and issues related to the case. Any questions asked should be written in the margins of the case logs, or on a separate sheet, together with the student's answers. By doing this, you will be able to confirm students' underpinning knowledge. If perhaps they have omitted to include some information, particularly within the first couple of case logs, this means of questioning enables students to provide sufficient evidence without having to rewrite the case log itself. Neither your students nor you have time to rewrite or reassess cases time after time. This is both demoralizing and unnecessary.

You must write by hand both your questions and your student's answers, your reflective comments and the date at the time of signing each case log. Such comments ensure the validity of the assessment and provide a more valuable record than perfectly drafted case logs. It is worth remembering that the portfolio is a working document and should show a natural progression throughout its completion, demonstrating the knowledge and experience your students have gained during their training.

○ Can I ask my student to add information to a case log?

● No, once a case log has been assessed, signed and dated, no amendments should be made to it. This is why assessment should be undertaken with the student so that questioning can be used to gain additional information.

○ *Is it possible to cross-reference cases within the portfolio?*

● Yes, this is strongly encouraged. The portfolio modules should be viewed as a whole and not isolated pieces of work. It may well be possible to cross-reference between several modules. For example, nursing of a single patient may provide evidence for laboratory, medical and fluid therapy, or perhaps radiography, surgical or anaesthesia case logs. Each case log must be completed, but where specific information relates to other modules the student can simply write in the case log reference number and page number in the relevant box(es).

○ *As an assessor must I write comments on all the case logs?*

● Yes. You are making a judgement on both your students' practical performance as well as the content of the case log and must include a reflective comment as evidence of their practical competence.

○ *Can supplementary evidence be included within a portfolio?*

● Any supplementary evidence must relate directly to work the student has carried out and be either photocopies of the original documents or, in the case of dispensing labels, additional copies produced at the time. You should ensure client confidentiality by crossing out name details, etc. In some modules, where additional evidence is required the guidance notes clearly state the type of supplementary evidence to include (e.g. consent forms, hospitalization charts, dispensing labels, anaesthesia charts, fluid therapy monitoring charts). Where other staff have also been involved in nursing a patient, your students should highlight their input on the relevant chart, or initial it to demonstrate the actual nursing care they carried out.

○ *Are module summary sheets necessary for each module?*

● Yes. As your students work through each module, you must check to ensure that the evidence they are producing meets the relevant Occupational Standards. On completion of a module you should write a reflective comment on their performance and progress during its completion and identify the types of evidence that have been generated (e.g. portfolio, questioning, etc.).

○ *Do I have to produce an assessment plan for every assessment?*

● No, the reality of working in practice means that you do not always have time to plan for every case your student wishes to include as evidence. However, by using the assessment planning and tutorial record annexe F, you can record what evidence is required and when your student plans to produce it. If, for instance, a student requires a radiograph using contrast media, then under 'action to be taken' you might state that the next myelogram that is admitted will be used as evidence. A target date can be written in and at the next tutorial you can confirm whether this has been met.

○ *How many students can an assessor mentor?*

● In a large training practice where there is more than one student and assessor, it is sensible to allocate specific students to specific assessors. A recommended ratio of assessor to students is 1 to 3, or a maximum of 1 to 2 where the assessor is unqualified.

○ *What if I don't get on with my assessor/my student?*

● The first thing is to determine what the actual problem is. We are all only human and have off days when things go from bad to worse and, possibly, may take things out of context. Therefore a misunderstanding may have arisen that can be sorted by the assessor and student talking things through. However, if they really feel unable to talk with each other, the internal verifier can help and should offer support. As a last resort, if there is a serious clash of personality between the student and the assessor, the only solution may be to reallocate the student with another assessor, and vice versa.

○ *Do I always have to produce written and oral questions with each assessment?*

● Yes and no! It is not necessary to produce a specified number of written and oral questions in the same way you did for your assessor training. Some assessments will only involve oral questioning, particularly where additional evidence is required to meet specific Occupational Standards, with your questions and your student's answers providing all the evidence. Even oral questions and answers have to be recorded, however, otherwise there is no actual evidence to demonstrate that the Occupational Standards have indeed been met. Questioning is usually necessary in relation to portfolio evidence; again both these and the answers should be recorded in the margin. It is not sufficient to write 'Student answered my questions correctly'.

○ *What can I do if I don't agree with my assessor's decision?*

● You should discuss this with your assessor first and hopefully this will clarify the decision. However, if you are still not happy you have the right to appeal. Each TP must have an appeals policy that identifies the means by which a student can appeal against an assessment decision. This document should be made available to all students and some practices actually display a copy on their student training board.

The Veterinary Nursing Approved Centre

Approved by the RCVS, Veterinary Nursing Approved Centres (VNACs) provide the necessary link between the awarding body and the Training and Assessment Practice. A centre may be a course provider (college), a very large veterinary hospital or a practice with several assessors and an internal verifier; alternatively, it may be a group of practices working together. The centre employs at least one IV, who visits practices on behalf of the RCVS to approve potential training and assessment practices and, when approved, to monitor their facilities, staffing levels, assessment decisions and the support provided to their students. Such visits form part of the VNAC's quality assurance mechanism. Where the centre is also a course provider, students attending their courses are often working in practices affiliated with the centre as a TP. However, a TP may have reason to send its students to a different college from the one to which it is affiliated. If a practice has several students, for instance, rather than lose them all on the same day it may seek course provision elsewhere.

ROLES AND RESPONSIBILITIES

The head of the centre is ultimately accountable to the RCVS and oversees the IVs within its team. Depending on the size of VNAC, the individual roles and responsibilities will depend on the number of staff employed and the time allocated for individual roles. In a small VNAC, the head of the centre and IV may be the same person.

The internal verifier

IVs must hold either the TDLB D34 internal verifier award or the Employment National Training Organization (ENTO) V1 unit. However, they do not have to hold either D32, 33 or A1. The Assessment Strategy stipulates that veterinary nurses or veterinary surgeons must have at least 2 years' postqualification experience in practice before embarking on IV training, and that they must occupy a position within the organization that gives them the authority and resources to carry out their role. This includes coordinating the work of assessors, providing training, advice and guidance, holding meetings, observing assessments in the workplace and internally verifying assessment decisions. Like all those involved with the veterinary nursing NVQ, they must be occupationally competent, fully conversant with the Occupational Standards and actively engage in relevant CPD.

An internal verifier must:

- be either a veterinary surgeon or listed veterinary nurse
- have 2 years' postqualification experience in practice before undertaking IV training
- hold either the D34 or V1 internal verifier award, or be working towards it
- undertake CPD.

V1 TRAINING

A trainee V1 internal verifier must provide evidence of supporting, monitoring and internally verifying the assessment decisions of two assessors.

The V1 unit is broken down into four elements:

V1.1 Carry out and evaluate internal assessment and quality assurance systems

V1.2 Support assessors

V1.3 Monitor the quality of assessors' performance

V1.4 Meet external quality assurance requirements.

Each element is broken down into performance criteria and, as with the A1 elements, these have been reworded in the following text to help you interpret their meaning. It is recommended that you read these together with the original copy supplied by your tutor.

V1.1

This involves the IV ensuring that the requirements of the A1 award are met by assessors in TPs and that they are involved with developing procedural documentation to ensure quality assurance, for both assessment and verification, and putting these into effect.

a. The IV should ensure that the VNAC IV sampling strategy and policy are put into practice to review assessment in affiliated TPs and verification within the centre, in line with RCVS requirements.

b. The IV should ensure that the sampling policy and strategy are based on the Occupational Standards for veterinary nursing.

c. Each year the RCVS undertakes a 'systems' audit and a 'portfolio' audit at each VNAC and visits random TPs affiliated with it. The IV will have to provide the relevant paperwork, tracking, reports, etc. to demonstrate your internal verification practice.

d. The centre's own internal verification policy will stipulate the level of support the IV provides to assessors and factors that influence any changes to this.

e. Every VNAC is required to hold standardization meetings for assessors within their affiliated TPs. Attendance records must be kept.

f. The IV should ensure that each TP has a complaints procedure and appeals policy and that the students are aware of it. A copy should be provided if necessary and any records relating to complaints or appeals should be kept.

g. Each VNAC must review and evaluate its own IV practice and act on external verifiers' reports.

h. In line with awarding body requirements and reports, the IV must identify potential changes to the centre's IV policy or strategy and ways of implementing them.

V1.2

This involves the IV providing support and guidance to assessors by observation and verification of assessment decisions.

a. In line with the Assessment Strategy, assessors must be either veterinary surgeons or nurses and have 2 year's postqualification experience before undertaking assessor training.

b. The IV should inform assessors of the evidence requirements for veterinary nursing and the relevant assessment documentation to use.

c. The IV should identify assessors' needs in terms of their knowledge and understanding of the assessment process, and encourage them to identify the needs of their students and how to maintain occupational competency through CPD.

d. The IV regularly observes and verifies assessment decisions in order to provide feedback to assessors on their assessment practice.

e. Each VNAC must provide standardization sessions to enable assessors to share assessment practice with others and discuss the outcomes.

f. The IV must observe each assessor's assessment decisions, verify different types of assessment evidence and check that assessors engage in relevant CPD in order to ensure individual assessment standards are maintained.

V1.3

This involves the IV observing assessors and verifying their assessment decisions.

a. The IV should look for evidence of assessment planning within the practice.

b. The IV should make sure that every assessor always uses the Occupational Standards when making an assessment decision.

c. Assessors must be able to determine whether the national standards have been met or not, and what action to take in each instance.

d. The IV should observe all assessors and look at the relevant paperwork in relation to all students being assessed by each, to confirm that individual assessors are applying safe, fair, valid and reliable methods of assessing candidates' competence.

e. Internally verifying assessors' assessment decisions over a period of time will enable the IV to look for evidence of consistency in their judgements. This will involve verifying a range of evidence and observing assessments within a TP.

f. A sampling strategy must include all assessors, all of the Occupational Standards and be done over a 5-year period to ensure that individual assessors are verified against all of the Occupational Standards.

g. To ensure consistency of assessment decisions within all TPs, the IV should visit different practices to observe the assessment therein and hold standardization meetings, which must be attended by a number of assessors from a range of practices.

h. Each time IVs visit a practice, they should interview students to ascertain the effectiveness of the assessor–student relationship.

i. While undertaking monitoring visits, the IV should confirm that health and safety and environmental protection procedures are being applied. In addition, discussion with students will confirm equal opportunities are being met.

j. The IV should check the relevant paperwork is being completed to demonstrate that assessors are carrying out reviews on their students' progress.

k. The IV should look for evidence of written and verbal feedback being recorded in the practice and discuss the feedback process with the students to determine it meets their needs.

l. Evidence of assessment records must be seen within the practice and all documentation must be kept confidential.

m. The IV should always provide assessors with constructive verbal and written feedback. A copy should be given to them and one kept for the IV's records.

V1.4

This involves the IV demonstrating an understanding of awarding body requirements for quality assurance. An internal verification policy and sampling strategy will provide evidence for this element.

a. A sampling strategy will demonstrate how an IV will be, or has been monitoring assessors' assessment decisions during a given year. It will include observation, verification of different types of evidence, interviews with students and assessors.

b. The IV should keep individual records for each assessor demonstrating which units and elements and which type of evidence have been verified and when the assessment was observed. In addition, copies of internal verification reports must be referred to in order to confirm that assessors are acting upon the advice in them.

c. The IV should give assessors written notice of when portfolio or other types of evidence are to be submitted for internal verification.

d. The IV should provide the RCVS external verifiers with any information they request on assessors, their students, etc.

e. The IV should answer any queries raised by RCVS external verifiers and provide written documentation as necessary.

f. If necessary, the IV should discuss any concerns about an external verification decision and ask for clarification. Any decision made by the external verifiers will be based on awarding body requirements in line with the Code of Practice.

g. The IV should seek guidance from the RCVS if a matter cannot be dealt with internally. This can be by phone, fax and email or in writing and copies of all correspondence should be kept.

h. The IV should always disseminate external verifier reports to assessors and confirm good and poor practice as necessary.

i. The IV should provide evidence to demonstrate that advice given by the external verifier has been acted upon.

In addition to demonstrating practical ability to internally verify and support assessors, as a trainee V1 internal verifier you will have to provide evidence of your underpinning knowledge of the nature and role of internal quality assurance of assessments, principles and concepts and external factors influencing internal quality assurance. The knowledge requirements will be given to you by your V1 tutor together with a list of questions. Your answers, if correct, will demonstrate your underpinning knowledge and provide the necessary evidence accordingly.

INTERNAL VERIFICATION

Often referred to as the 'guardian of the standards', the IV is responsible for ensuring that all assessments carried out within TPs meet the National Occupational Standards. As such, it is a role that is vital to the integrity of the veterinary nursing NVQ. To be effective, as an IV you must demonstrate the following practice:

- provide appropriate training and support to the assessor team
- regularly monitor the work of each assessor and the quality of assessment
- provide feedback on assessment decisions
- ensure adequate assessment resources are available
- keep accurate records
- liaise with the external verifiers
- monitor professional and occupational competence of assessors, as well as their own.

TP APPROVAL AND MONITORING

All potential training and assessment practices must have an approval visit by an IV to confirm that the practice has the necessary facilities, resources and workload to support veterinary nursing training. On receipt of the application form from a potential TP, as the IV you should take a close look at it and make a note of whether there are any gaps or areas that you need to clarify. It may be that a phone call to the principal or assessor is all that is needed to confirm something prior to your visit. If you work as part of a team of IVs, you can always discuss issues with colleagues; alternatively you may wish to ring the RCVS and seek guidance or clarification from the centre approval officer.

The initial visit to the practice is likely to take 1 to 2 hours depending on its size and the number of students and assessors. You need to meet all the staff involved in assessment and see the facilities relating to the training of nurses. It is important to remember that the emphasis is on the training and support of students. The approval criteria have been stipulated to ensure that students have access to fair and reliable assessment within the veterinary practice. Remember that you are undertaking the approval visit on behalf of the RCVS and ultimately the decision as to whether a practice can be approved as a TP lies with this body. Your role as IV is to make a recommendation for approval, which is based on the criteria within the application form and backed up with a completed IV visit report, with action points identified and agreed with the principal where necessary. If you are unsure about any aspect of the approval system, you should telephone the RCVS, which will be happy to advise you.

The comprehensive report, supplied by the RCVS, is completed by the IV and includes details of staff, facilities, clinical workload, equipment, library books, etc. In conjunction with the head of centre, the IV is responsible for ensuring that adequate assessment resources are available for each student veterinary nurse as well as assuring the overall quality of training and assessment. This is undertaken in the first instance through the approval system of the TP and monitored closely by maintaining constant contact with and by holding up-to-date records in respect of individual TPs. A change of staff within a TP can have a huge impact on the assessment process and the IV must ensure students always have access to reliable training and assessment.

Approval can be granted for a maximum of 5 years, with an annual review being undertaken by the VNAC to ensure that TP status can be continued. Many prospective TPs have action points that need addressing and the principal and IV will agree these, together with a date for resolution; approval being held pending a satisfactory response. The visit also enables the IV to determine the level of support needed for assessors within each TP. New assessors will require a structured induction; some VNACs also provide assessor training. Trainee assessors must have their assessment decisions countersigned either by another, qualified, assessor, usually one within the TP, or by an IV. If the latter, a different IV will then have to verify the assessor's decisions internally, as it is not acceptable to verify a judgement you have been involved with. By providing the TPs with their contact details, IVs can ensure that guidance and support may be sought as necessary. A memorandum of agreement is signed by both the principal of the TP and the head of centre of the VNAC. Principals need not be assessors themselves and it is essential that they sign the agreement to demonstrate their commitment and compliance to the scheme. This agreement outlines the VNAC's provision for internal verification, contact details and response times and the commitment of the practice to the assessment and training of students and attendance at meetings held by the VNAC. Attendance by assessors at these meetings is mandatory as these will include CPD activities such as standardization sessions along with updates on developments within the veterinary industry, the VN awards and Occupational Standards.

Following approval, at least two further visits to a TP will be undertaken each year. During visits every assessor will be observed carrying out a practical assessment with a student and monitoring of facilities and staffing levels will also take place. IVs may wish to take a checklist with them, which can then be referred to when writing up the report of the visit. During a monitoring visit it is important to include the following:

- *practice facilities and equipment* – the IV should tour the practice to confirm no changes have occurred that would affect TP status
- *confirm caseloads* – clinical, surgical and radiography
- *interview students and assessors* – check the rota for any changes that may impact on training and assessment
- *inspect paperwork* – minutes of staff meetings, equipment maintenance records, student portfolio, assessment plans, tracking documents, etc.

Internal verification sampling of portfolios may take place during a TP visit, but portfolios will also be called into the VNAC for verification. Additional visits by the IV may be deemed necessary to support unqualified or inexperienced assessors, or if any problems are identified.

The centre must hold a file for each TP containing the following type of information:

- details about each assessor:
  - curriculum vitae demonstrating occupational competence
  - original D32/33 or A1 certificates must be seen and authenticated copies kept (i.e. where an IV signs and dates the back of the photocopy)
  - CPD undertaken (copies of certificates of attendance, etc.)
  - annual verification of RCVS listing (veterinary nurses) and registration (veterinary surgeons)
- copies of all correspondence between the centre and TP, including telephone calls and contact via email
- IV reports in respect of TP approval and monitoring visits
- IV reports on assessment verification, both sampling and final
- TP risk banding, including any measures being implemented to reduce the level of risk where necessary
- student details, including evidence of interviews during monitoring visits.

UNQUALIFIED ASSESSORS

Where an assessor within one of the TPs is working towards the assessor award, it is essential that you as IV determine a realistic target date for

Figure 4.1 Assessor observation report.

Assessor:	A Nurse		Student:	A Student
TP:	A Veterinary Surgery		Date:	

Assessment task:	Prepare the necessary equipment and position the 'sedated dog' for an X-ray of its pelvis for the Kennel Club Hip Dysplasia Scheme.

Unit and elements:	Unit 9 9.1 9.2 9.3	Module:	8

Simulation	✔	Observation of set tasks:	✔	Written evidence		Questioning	✔ 9.3

	Assessor action	Internal verifier's comments
1.	Agreed assessment with the student and explained process	Assessment agreed in advance and assessor discussed it at the time of the assessment in my presence.
2.	Student aware of occupational standards and evidence requirements	Assessor clearly explained the assessment task, the signed plan stated the units and elements being covered. This task was a simulation using a toy dog in preparation for the level 3 practical exams.
3.	Put the student at ease	Yes.
4.	Asked relevant, clear questions	Yes. Where further clarification was required, the assessor was able to elicit this by rewording a question.
5.	Gave appropriate feedback as soon as practicable	Yes. The assessor was very encouraging and told the student at each stage how well they had done. When a question was incorrectly answered, the assessor gave the correct answer.
6.	Encouraged the student to self-assess performance and ask questions	A good relationship between student and assessor was demonstrated. This allowed for discussion when the student was either unsure about a question or unable to answer it.
7.	Further action agreed with student where necessary	Student very competent at task but requested more practice at collimation. It was agreed that she will be involved with as many genuine radiography cases leading up to the exams as is practical. Additional simulation may also be used.
8.	Assessment decision recorded. Evidence requirements met and recorded	Yes, the assessor used photocopies of the occupational standards and recorded all answers and decisions on these. Student and assessor signed documentation.
9.	Assessor's self-assessment and comments:	

I feel the assessment went well, Anne is clearly very competent at radiography positioning but needs to gain in confidence especially with describing anatomical landmarks.

continued overpage

Figure 4.1 – continued

10.	Internal verifier's comments and recommendations:
	Sarah demonstrated excellent assessment skills in her planning, helping to make her student feel at ease and in her questioning technique. By giving feedback all the way through she helped give Anne confidence and when Anne was unable to answer a question she provided discussion and clarification. We discussed how a different questioning technique may be required for less confident students who may not be happy to answer questions as they perform a task. This can put some students off and may also make them lose track of the task itself.

Internal verifier:	VN/MRCVS
Signature:	Date:

achieving certification. You must monitor the trainee's progress and ensure that any assessment decisions are validated by a qualified assessor, either within the TP or if necessary from within the VNAC. In order to authenticate the trainee assessor's decision, you must observe the person assessing and have a range of assessment practice sampled, involving different types of evidence (e.g. written questions, portfolio case logs, essays, etc.). Remember that as the IV you cannot be involved with verifying an assessment decision you yourself have made or validated.

It is strongly recommended that trainee assessors attend all meetings and workshops provided by their VNAC. This will ensure they have opportunities to discuss assessment techniques, and alternative assessment methods, and are kept informed of awarding body requirements and updates. Figure 4.1 is an example of an assessor observation report; it is an amended version of the one provided by the RCVS in the Centre Handbook.

Monitoring and review of student progress will involve the IV looking closely at the following aspects:

- *theoretical training* – where are students attending college, and does the TP have a copy of the scheme of work and any student reports?
- *student/assessor rota* – does the assessor have time allocated to carry out the role?
- *tutorials* – how regularly are these being held and are they being recorded?
- *staff meetings* – who attends, are they held regularly and are minutes kept?
- *IV/assessor meetings* – where there is more than one assessor in a TP, are they holding formal or informal meetings, and are the assessors attending your VNAC workshops?
- *validation of assessment decisions by IV*:
  - observation of practical assessment
  - portfolio sampling
  - other evidence (e.g. questioning, essays, etc.)
- *CPD by students and assessors* – are copies of attendance being kept for all relevant CPD attended?

VERIFYING ASSESSMENT DECISIONS

The sampling strategy

A sampling strategy must be devised by the IV, who will need to identify the risk assessment rating of each TP. The strategy will be based on this and the following information:

- *the number and location of the TPs* – this has a bearing on the IV's time; also check whether an assessor works at more than one TP
- *the experience of the assessor(s)* – inexperienced assessors may not be familiar with the standards and assessment methods; the sample should include a larger proportion of their assessment decisions than those of experienced assessors
- *the number of assessors*:
  - all assessors must be included in the sample
  - time allocated for assessor role; check the rota
- *the number of and NVQ level of students* – a range of students within both level 2 and level 3 must be included in the sample
- *the Occupational Standards within the NVQ* – some elements may have extensive range statements, or be more difficult to provide evidence for or to assess
- *the range of assessment methods* – these should include observation, portfolio, questioning, witness statements, simulation, professional discussion, projects, etc.

The VNAC's sampling strategy stipulates how often the IV will visit the practice; it is usually at least twice each year. One visit will be to observe assessors; the other will be a monitoring visit where facilities and human resources are checked. Students should be interviewed during each visit. Depending on the outcome of a monitoring visit or verification of assessment decisions, it may be necessary to increase the number of visits or amount of evidence sampled. As an IV you are effectively reviewing your sampling strategy based on any changes to the assessor team, the practice facilities or the standards of assessment decisions. Such reviews are essential to ensure that you provide the appropriate level of support and guidance. Where necessary you may have to stipulate action to be taken or impose sanctions to ensure that assessments continue to be fair, reliable, valid, sufficient and current.

It is a requirement that the VNAC's sampling strategy works across all units and elements. It must include a representative sample of assessment decisions and candidate evidence to ensure that decisions are being made only against the Occupational Standards and are fair, accurate and reliable.

Sampling of assessments must include both interim and summative sampling. Interim sampling is where the IV looks at the assessment process at different stages of the evidence being collected and assessed. It should involve reviewing students' work during planning, review and completion; it will therefore entail checking how the assessor discusses and gives feedback to students on their progress as well as the effectiveness of assessment planning. Summative sampling involves reviewing the quality of the assessment decisions and how these were reached. An IV must be able to identify through the sampling that the assessor has checked whether the evidence has met the Occupational Standards.

A sampling grid is a useful tool for IVs to record their results on each time they verify an assessor, either by directly observing them assessing in practice or by sampling different types of assessment evidence. Figure 4.2 is an example of an assessment-sampling grid. This document could be used either for one assessor only or to record verification of different assessors within a TP. Documented evidence of IV sampling and reports must be kept in respect of individual TPs and assessors both at the VNAC and the TP.

Assessment verification must consist of the following three activities to ensure that assessment is consistent and reliable across all TPs:

- observing assessments
- sampling assessment decisions
- standardizing assessment judgements.

Observing assessments

Each assessor must be observed working with a candidate on at least one occasion a year (i.e. every 6 to 12 months). Trainee and inexperienced assessors (i.e. within 1 year of their gaining D32, 33 or A1 assessor awards) will need more frequent monitoring and support than experienced assessors. As well as observing the assessment process, the IV will need to see evidence of documentation within each TP to demonstrate that the assessors are planning assessments, holding regular tutorial sessions, and providing oral and written feedback to their students, and that the interpersonal skills needed to support students are evident. It is essential to interview students also to ensure that they understand the assessment and appeal processes and to determine whether they have confidence in their assessor. All assessment documentation relating to students must be kept confidentially in a locked cupboard or drawer within the TP.

Sampling assessment decisions

A range of evidence types must be included, although the portfolio will constitute the bulk of evidence. Sampling must take place during the collection of evidence and compilation of the portfolio at each level and again once all the evidence has been completed, prior to certification being applied for. It is important to remember, when sampling, that one or two case logs cannot provide sufficient evidence to meet the required standards in terms of practical competence, underpinning knowledge and scope or range for specific units or elements. Therefore students are very likely to have to provide additional evidence by answering the assessor's

Figure 4.2 Example assessment-sampling grid.

INTERNAL VERIFICATION OF ASSESSMENT SAMPLING GRID

Internal verifier: *Jill Warner* Year of sampling: *2004*

Name of TP: *A Veterinary Surgery*

TP no: *100000*

Assessor	Date of sampling	Student/ NVQ Level	Unit: 7	Unit: 8	Unit: 9	Unit: 10	Unit: 11	Unit: 12	Unit: 13	Observation of set tasks	Simulation	Written evidence	Questioning/ testing
A Vet	24.01.04	AB Level 3	✓	✓	✓	✓						P	✓
A Nurse	24.01.04	BC Level 3				✓	✓	✓				P	
A Nurse	13.02.04	BC Level 3	✓		✓					✓			✓
A Vet	06.03.04	AB Level 3	✓							✓			✓
A Vet	15.05.04	AB Level 3		✓		✓	✓					P	✓
A Nurse	15.05.04	BC Level 3	✓	✓				✓				P	✓

Units sampled / Assessment type

INTERNAL VERIFICATION OF ASSESSMENT SAMPLING GRID

Internal verifier:

Year of sampling:

Name of TP:

TP no:

Assessor	Date of sampling	Student/ NVQ Level	Units sampled								Assessment type				
			Unit: CU2	Unit: CU5	Unit: 1	Unit: 2	Unit: 3	Unit: 4	Unit: 5	Unit: 6	Unit: 7	Observation of set tasks	Simulation	Written evidence	Questioning/ testing

oral/written questions correctly and via the appropriate use of simulation, particularly when clinical skills are being assessed.

All evidence must be:

- *reliable* – reflect a level of performance consistently demonstrated by students in their work
- *valid* – relevant to the veterinary nursing Occupational Standards
- *sufficient* – meet all the requirements of the standards in full
- *current* – recent enough to be certain that the student retains the previous level of skill, understanding and knowledge and reflects ongoing assessment
- *authentic* – have been produced by the student in question and relate to genuine cases; as IV you may well ask to see client records while sampling assessment evidence.

As an IV you must take care to avoid reassessing (second-assessing) as there can be a temptation when internally (or externally) verifying to take on the role of the assessor. Remember that your role here is rather to *validate* assessment practice and decisions.

Standardizing assessment judgements

It will be necessary to review assessment planning regularly to ensure that assessments within each TP are fair, accurate, consistent and valid. Where possible, the work of different assessors within a TP should be compared across the same units to confirm that they are assessing to the same level. It is equally important to ensure that the requirements of the National Occupational Standards are not either being exceeded by overenthusiastic assessors or not being met by insufficient evidence being generated. Regular meetings with groups of assessors provide opportunities to undertake standardization exercises and to demonstrate examples of good practice.

Where a VNAC has more than one IV, peer review and standardization sessions within the IV team are essential to ensure their verification decisions and judgements remain consistent. Regular attendance at RCVS IV meetings is mandatory to ensure that all IVs are kept up to date with awarding body requirements, current changes within the VN award and related documentation.

EXAMPLE IV REPORTS

The RCVS has provided sample documentation at the back of the Centre Handbook. Alternatively you may already have access to IV reports, or wish to devise your own. You may prefer to have two different forms, using one for interim sampling and one as a final IV report. The first example included here is based on the RCVS report (Fig. 4.3) and the second is a slightly modified report (Fig. 4.4).

EXAMPLE IV REPORTS • 135

Figure 4.3 Example RCVS report.

Student name:		A Student		NVQ level	2 ✔	3
Assessor name:		An Assessor		TDLB D32/33	Y ✔	N
Training and assessment practice:		A Veterinary Practice				

Units sampled	Unit/Element complete Yes / No	Comments	Assessor actions	Actions met/date
Units CU2 and CU5	Yes	Unit supported with witness testimonies as per guidelines.		
Units VN1 and VN5	Partially	Although portfolio guidance has been met, the occupational standards require cats, dogs and exotics. Therefore additional evidence is required for Unit 5 element 5.4 'provide veterinary materials to clients' scope exotics.		
Unit VN6	Yes	Excellent use of witness statements to confirm advice clearly given to clients.		
Unit VN2	Yes	Species range met for admission and discharge of patients.		
Units VN3 and VN4	Yes	Good range of cases and species to meet occupational standards.		
Personal profile and employment record	Yes			
Authentication sheet	Yes			
Planning form/grid	Yes			
Assessor summary sheets	Yes	In respect of completed modules/units		

Summary comments:

You clearly demonstrate your understanding of the assessment process. The use of further questioning throughout the case logs and as additional assessments has ensured that most of the occupational standards have been met. However, Unit 5 element 5.4 'provide veterinary materials to clients' scope – an exotic has not been included. Please confirm whether you have evidence at the surgery for this or if not, ensure that Anne produces some.

Overall standard of evidence:		Satisfactory	✔	Unsatisfactory	
Portfolio complete (Applicable only on final verification for award)		Yes		No	

Name of internal verifier:	Jill Warner		VN or MRCVS No:	VN 6002068
Signature:			Date:	

Figure 4.4 Example modified interim report.

Date	11.02.04	Report no.	3
Candidate name	A Student	Training practice	A Veterinary Surgery
Enrolment number	E2004	TP Number	01020304
Assessor name	An Assessor	Assessor qualifications	D32,33
Units/modules verified	Overall verification of Level 2 portfolio to assess student progress and action taken following previous IV report of 28.01.04		

Feedback for assessor:

Comments made in previous IV report have been duly addressed.
    Excellent use of assessor questioning throughout portfolio. Witness statements used in support of cases.
    Appendices 1, 2, 3, 4 & 5 submitted. However, 6 and 7 have been omitted. These must be internally verified at next submission or during next IV visit to practice on 2 Mar

The following cases need to be completed:
    Module 1
    1a × 1
    1b × 1

    Module 2
    2c × 2

    Module 3
    3a × 1
    3b × 2
    Module 4
    Complete
    Module 5
    5a × 1
    5b × 1
    5c × 1 intravenous injection.

National Standards Met:	Yes No ✔ further evidence required
Internal verifier signature	
Internal verifier name/qualifications	Jill Warner
Date of signature	

STANDARDIZATION OF ASSESSMENT PRACTICE

Standardization of assessment practice is undertaken to ensure that all candidates in a TP are assessed fairly and to give credibility to the assessment system. Where there is more than one student in a TP, as IV you should ensure that all are given the opportunity to produce the evidence they need. There is a temptation when one of the students is enthusiastic for the assessor to concentrate on this student, particularly if another has to be coerced into being assessed and writing up the case logs.

It is also your role as IV to ensure that all assessments carried out within affiliated TPs meet the requirements of the National Occupational Standards. This is achieved by each IV ensuring that the appropriate evidence is gathered by the students in the first place, by auditing the evidence to check it links to the Occupational Standards and by improving consistency of assessment decisions between assessors. When looking at the assessment decisions of each assessor, there must be evidence to demonstrate that the assessor observed the student perform the task, that further questioning has taken place to confirm underpinning knowledge and that a full range of strategies has been used to meet the different units within the Occupational Standards.

The performance of the IV is in turn monitored by the EV, who provides oral and written feedback on the systems used and the verification carried out. It is a vital role of IVs to disseminate the EV reports and use them as a tool for improvement, both of their own practice and of the assessors in their affiliated TPS.

The role of the head of centre is to ensure that:

- there is a cohesive IV team who meet regularly and attend meetings held by the awarding body
- the record keeping within the centre is comprehensive and up to date for each TP, with current and relevant information on its assessors and students
- risk banding of individual TPs is carried out and monitored regularly with the appropriate level of support being provided to the practice
- validation of assessment decisions can be confirmed
- support is provided to the IVs in terms of time, CPD, etc., and to the associated TPs.

CLAIMING FOR CERTIFICATION

The veterinary nursing NVQ consists of two levels, within which are eight units for level 2 and seven units for level 3 (see Ch. 2, Tables 2.1 and 2.2). On completion of all the units for each level, a student also has to undergo the RCVS independent assessments (multiple choice papers and also practical examinations for level 3). On passing these examinations and having their portfolio verified as meeting the national standard, the head of centre of the VNAC puts in a claim for NVQ certification from the RCVS. At level 3, a student is also awarded a certificate in either small animal or equine veterinary nursing.

Students are also eligible to claim for individual unit certification, which literally means that, on completing an entire NVQ unit and producing the required evidence, a claim can be put in to the RCVS and a certificate issued confirming which unit has been awarded. This certificate remains valid for 5 years, after which a student would have to produce new, current evidence of practical competence and underpinning knowledge. Where a student takes time out of training for a period of time, this enables credit to be awarded for previous experience and abilities. Unit credit can also be claimed when a student moves from one TP to another that is affiliated with a different VNAC. This can be helpful for the assessor in the new practice, who can then be assured that any previously assessed evidence has definitely met the national standards.

EVALUATION

As with all aspects of teaching, assessment and verification, the VNAC must demonstrate that TPs have undergone self-evaluation and subsequently made appropriate changes where necessary. As IV you should provide your TPs with an evaluation form or questionnaire, which can be completed confidentially if a TP wishes. Which person in the TP should complete the form will depend on whether principals are involved with assessment and training themselves. If not, it would be more appropriate for assessors to give their feedback.

The form should always include a space for the name of the TP and a signatory as it is essential to identify where an individual problem or dissatisfaction exists. An evaluation questionnaire should include questions to confirm that:

■ details are provided of who the IV is and how to contact the person

■ queries from TPs are being dealt with efficiently and effectively

■ current awarding body information is being disseminated to all assessors

■ appropriate guidance and support are being given, particularly to unqualified assessors

■ visits are being planned in advance, and appropriate notice is given with an explanation of any paperwork required

■ oral and written feedback is provided at the end of all visits

■ a written report is sent following a visit.

Figure 4.5 is an example of an IV/assessor support form that may beused.

FREQUENTLY ASKED QUESTIONS AND ANSWERS

○ *How can I become an IV?*

● Veterinary nurses or veterinary surgeons must have at least 2 years' postqualification experience in practice before embarking on training to be an IV, and must occupy a position within the organization that gives them the authority and resources to carry out their role. In the future it may become a requirement that applicants have first achieved either the TDLB D32 and 33 or A1 awards.

Figure 4.5 IV/assessor support form.

Internal verifier: ....

Assessor: ....

I confirm that the internal verifier has:

Provided me with full, up-to-date awarding body documentation records and guidelines ☐

Given me accurate advice and support to enable me to identify and meet my training and development needs ☐

Provided accurate advice concerning the appropriate and efficient use of different types of evidence ☐

Assisted me with arrangements for candidates with special assessment requirement ☐

Allocated responsibilities to me that are clear and match the needs of students and myself ☐

Provided me with accurate, up-to-date advice and relevant support to achieve consistency in assessments ☐

I hold the assessor award(s)   D32 ☐   D33 ☐   A1 ☐

I am working towards the award(s)   D32 ☐   D33 ☐   A1 ☐

Signed: .... (Assessor)   Date: ....

Name of TP: ....

○ *Once qualified, who supports and monitors me?*

● The RCVS as the awarding body appoints external verifiers. These support and monitor the internal verifiers by providing telephone and email contact, initially approving the VNACs and visiting at least twice each year to monitor their systems and sample verification decisions. Support is also provided by holding workshops where IVs are kept up to date on awarding body and industry issues.

○ *How often should I verify a student's portfolio?*

● A minimum of twice at each level; once during compilation and once on completion. This will depend on the qualification and experience of the assessor involved, however. If the person is unqualified or inexperienced, you must increase the sampling rate. Similarly, if you have concerns during the initial sampling, you should request the portfolio for additional sampling and not wait until its completion.

○ *Can an unqualified assessor sign off case logs in the portfolio?*

● Trainee assessors working towards their D32, 33 or A1 award can sign the case logs; however, another qualified assessor must countersign, having first observed the person assessing, to validate their decision.

○ *Can I countersign case logs for an unqualified assessor and then internally verify the portfolio?*

● No, you cannot verify your own assessment decisions. By countersigning for another trainee assessor, you would be doing just that.

○ *As an IV how many assessors can I be a verifier for?*

● Ultimately the awarding body decides this by approving the VNAC and monitoring the work of IVs. Its decision will depend on the experience and qualifications of the IV, the number of TPs affiliated with the VNAC and where they are located, the number and experience of the assessors, the number of students within each TP and how much time IVs are allocated to do their job.

○ *Is it possible to be allocated an alternative EV?*

● If you have a problem in respect of the EV you have been allocated, this should be discussed with the head of veterinary nursing at the RCVS. Alternative arrangements can be made if a good working relationship cannot be maintained.

○ *Can students work on other case logs while their portfolio is with the VNAC?*

● Yes, both student and TP should have a copy of the tracking documentation and tutorial records, which will confirm those cases that have yet to be completed. Not having the portfolio itself for a few days or weeks will not disadvantage the student, who can simply work on other cases.

○ *Does a student have to meet all the Occupational Standards?*

● Yes. When the veterinary nursing NVQ first came into being in January 1999, it was accepted that a student would be able to meet all the Occupational Standards by completing the portfolio, and passing the multiple choice exams and the practical exams. However, as the NVQ has developed, the RCVS now stipulate that all the units must be met within the evidence produced solely in practice. This has huge implications in terms of being able to cover the scope practically within the Occupational Standards. As such, questioning, additional assessments and the use of simulation as well as the portfolio evidence is likely to be needed to ensure all units are met.

External Organizations

THE AWARDING BODY: THE RCVS

The external verifier

The RCVS, as the awarding body for the veterinary nursing NVQ, appoints external verifiers who provide the link between the VNACs and the awarding body itself. An EV must hold either the TDLB D35 external verification award or the ENTO V2 unit. The VN Assessment Strategy stipulates that a veterinary nurse or veterinary surgeon must have 5 years' postqualification experience in the industry before becoming an EV. As with assessors and internal verifiers, EVs must ensure they maintain their occupational competence, and remain up to date with the latest developments within the industry and the NVQ system. To achieve the V2 unit an EV must 'conduct internal quality assurance of the assessment process'. The V2 unit is broken down into four elements:

V2.1 Monitor the internal quality assurance process

V2.2 Verify the quality of assessment

V2.3 Provide information, advice and support on the internal quality assurance of assessment processes

V2.3 Evaluate the effectiveness of external quality assurance of the assessment process.

The EVs have been allocated areas of responsibility geographically and are responsible for the VNACs within their own area. They are responsible in the first instance for undertaking the approval visit to each VNAC. They need to develop and maintain excellent working relationships with the staff in VNACs in order to be able to provide feedback on their verification practice, including any constructive criticism and negotiation of future action points. EVs' knowledge of the occupational standards and awarding body systems is essential to ensure that consistent advice and guidance are provided nationally to all VNACs. This is

An external verifier must:

- be either a veterinary surgeon or a listed veterinary nurse
- have a minimum of 5 years' postqualification experience
- hold either the D35 or V2 assessor award or be working towards it
- undertake CPD.

achieved by holding regular team meetings and liaising closely with each other and the awarding body itself. Although employed by the RCVS, EVs also have a responsibility to the Qualification and Curriculum Authority (QCA) to ensure the quality and credibility of the NVQ framework.

VNAC approval and monitoring visits

On receipt of the application form, the centre approval officer at the RCVS goes through the documentation before arranging for an EV to carry out an approval visit. During the visit the centre must demonstrate that it has the necessary staffing levels and systems in place to be able to monitor and support the prospective TPs, to ensure that standards of training and assessment are maintained. Approval may be given outright, or an action plan agreed with the head of centre and an appropriate date for resolution set.

Monitoring visits to the VNAC will be undertaken in respect of portfolio sampling and systems monitoring; this will involve a minimum of two visits per year. In addition, an EV will visit TPs affiliated with each VNAC and observe the IVs undertaking their role. Any decisions made by an EV are directly related to the Code of Practice that is produced by QCA. Where recommendations are made by an EV, it is the VNAC's responsibility to produce an action plan confirming how it is going to deal with any non-compliance that has been identified.

Dissemination of awarding body requirements

The RCVS endeavours to ensure that those working within the veterinary industry are kept informed of current issues. This is achieved via the RCVS website www.rcvs.org.uk, on which can be found all matters relating to veterinary nurse training and assessment, together with a list of VNACs and TPs, EV details and information on work-based assessment, examinations and postqualification RCVS awards (e.g. diplomas). Copies of the portfolio case logs, guidance notes, occupational standards and syllabus can be downloaded for use.

The EV team holds regular meetings for IVs across the country, for which annual attendance is mandatory. These meetings are an ideal way for verifiers to share experiences, both good and bad. Individual EVs are contactable by phone, email and fax either at home or via the RCVS.

Maintaining occupational competence

It is essential that those working as internal or external verifiers undertake clinical experience as part of their regular CPD. This will enable them to remain up to date on all issues relating to nursing in terms of facilities, materials, equipment, etc.

THE QUALIFICATION AND CURRICULUM AUTHORITY

The Qualification and Curriculum Authority (QCA) oversees the work of the RCVS as the awarding body for the veterinary nursing NVQ, to ensure that its administration, marketing and awarding procedures run efficiently. The QCA is sponsored by the Department for Education and Skills (DfES). The Secretary of State for Education and Skills appoints members to the board of governors who have experience in education, training and business. The QCA is responsible for accrediting and monitoring qualifications in colleges and at work, together with maintaining and developing the national curriculum and associated assessments, tests and examinations. The needs of employers and learners are met within the national qualifications framework. The QCA is able to accredit qualifications at appropriate levels and regularly review the suitability and availability of qualifications.

The NVQ Code of Practice

This document, together with the Common Code of Practice, specifies the quality assurance and control requirements that apply to all NVQs. The RCVS, as the awarding body, and the VNACs are responsible for ensuring that the management, administration, assessment and quality assurance for the veterinary nursing NVQ are consistent with the regulations set out in both documents. To this end, any enquiry or decision made in respect of approval of VNACs or TPs, candidate registration and certification, internal and external verification, sanctions for non-compliance, malpractice and appeals is based on the Code of Practice. This ensures the high quality and consistency of the standards in the assessment and awarding of the veterinary nursing NVQ.

LANTRA

Lantra is the Sector Skills Council for the environmental and land-based sector. It is an employer-led organization, licensed by government to represent the interests of businesses and employees of 17 industries, of which veterinary nursing is one. Following consultation with our industry they have produced the Assessment Strategy and National Occupational Standards for level 2 and level 3 veterinary nursing.

FREQUENTLY ASKED QUESTIONS AND ANSWERS

○ *How can I become an EV?*
● By being a qualified veterinary surgeon or listed veterinary nurse with 5 years' postqualification experience within the industry and holding either the TDLB D35 or the ENTO V2 award.

○ *Do verification decisions made by an unqualified EV have to be countersigned?*
● Yes, in exactly the same way as a trainee assessor or IV, another EV acts as a mentor and ensures the validity of the verification decisions.

○ *As an EV, how many centres can I be responsible for?*

● This will depend on the number of hours you are employed for by the awarding body and your experience and qualifications. In addition, the size and location of the VNACs and number of IVs and affiliated TPs will be taken into account.

○ *How is an EV monitored and by whom?*

● Quality assurance is monitored by the RCVS as the awarding body, which in turn is monitored by QCA. Peer reviews enable EVs to observe each other while undertaking approval and monitoring visits and when making subsequent decisions. Sampling of verification decisions relating to other sources of evidence (e.g. portfolio case logs) is also undertaken by the awarding body.

Developments in the Veterinary Nursing Profession

In the twenty-first century the emphasis is very much on the need for veterinary nursing to receive the professional status and recognition that it deserves. In order to do this, it has been agreed that we must become self-regulating and accountable for ourselves as nurses. As we move towards this goal, firstly by the implementation of voluntary regulation, there is the exciting prospect of veterinary nurses being able to develop their skills and qualifications further and to embrace the role of nurse fully within whichever veterinary practice they work. The needs of both the nurses and the industry must be continually reviewed and should be considered in unison rather than opposition.

VOCATIONALLY RELATED QUALIFICATIONS

In July 2003 the VN syllabus and independent assessments (external examinations) were accredited as Vocationally Related Qualifications (VRQs). This was necessary in order to provide a Technical Certificate, which will be a requirement if the veterinary industry introduces a Modern Apprenticeship framework in England as in Scotland. Both the syllabus and examinations remain essential to the veterinary nursing NVQ awards and all students must therefore complete them in order to achieve the level 2 and level 3 NVQ. As of September 2004, all course providers must be approved by the RCVS to ensure effective course provision. This involves ensuring there are suitably qualified teaching staff, and adequate classroom accommodation, library resources and teaching aids/resources to support students. The students will register for the VRQ awards via their veterinary nursing course provider (VNCP), which will provide the name, enrolment number and date of NVQ enrolment for each student. Candidates must be registered in order to enter the independent assessments and principals of the VNCPs will have to authorize their students' examination applications. Students must have achieved certification for level 2 before going on to a level 3 course. The deadline dates for registering students with the RCVS are between 1 September and 28 February in the relevant academic year.

CHOICE OF COURSE OR SPECIALISM

All nurses want to have the opportunity of progression and job satisfaction and be able to fulfil their ambitions. For several years now, there has been a choice of courses and a range of qualifications, including:

- VN certificate
  - equine
  - small animal
- HND
- degree – Foundation and Honours
- specialist top-up certificates
- diplomas in both surgical and medical nursing and dermatology
- schedule 3 – in which nurses are able to utilize their skills further, but must have the relevant qualifications and experience before undertaking additional tasks. Student nurses are able to undertake procedures to gain the experience and competence required.

Following the introduction of TPs and the implementation of the RCVS Practice Standards Tier System, standardization between practices generally, and especially those wishing to train veterinary nurses, will continue to be implemented and monitored. The bottom line is that all veterinary nurses want to have their skills recognized and utilized, and to reach their full potential as nurses within veterinary practice.

List of Abbreviations

A1	Unit qualification to assess candidates using a range of methods
A2	Unit qualification to assess candidates' performance through observation
ANA	Animal Nursing Assistant
ATAC	Approved Training and Assessment Centre
BSAVA	British Small Animal Veterinary Association
BVNA	British Veterinary Nursing Association
CPD	Continuing professional development
CU	Common unit
D32	Unit qualification to assess candidate performance
D33	Unit qualification to assess candidate using differing sources of evidence
DfES	Department for Education and Skills
ENTO	Employment National Training Organization
EV	External verifier
IV	Internal verifier
MCQ	Multiple choice question
NOS	National occupational standards
NVQ	National Vocational Qualification
PC	Performance criteria
QCA	Qualifications and Curriculum Authority
RANA	Registered Animal Nursing Auxiliary
RCVS	Royal College of Veterinary Surgeons
RTA	Road traffic accident
S/NVQ	Scottish and National Vocational Qualification
SVN	Student veterinary nurse
TDLB	Training and Development Lead Body
TP	Training and Assessment Practice
V1	Unit qualification to conduct internal quality assurance of the assessment process
V2	Unit qualification to conduct external quality assurance of the assessment process
VN	Veterinary nurse
VNAC	Veterinary Nursing Approved Centre
VNCP	Veterinary Nursing Course Provider
VRQ	Vocationally Related Qualification

Further Reading and Useful Websites

External Verification of NVQs: A guide for external verifiers.
  QCA Publications, PO Box 99, Sudbury, Suffolk, CO10 2SN.

Internal Verification of NVQs: A guide for internal verifiers.
  QCA Publications, PO Box 99, Sudbury, Suffolk, CO10 2SN.

Joint Awarding Body Guidance on Internal Verification of NVQs.
  QCA Publications, PO Box 99, Sudbury, Suffolk, CO10 2SN.

NVQ Code of Practice 2001.
  QCA Publications, PO Box 99, Sudbury, Suffolk, CO10 2SN.

Useful websites:

www.rcvs.org.uk

www.qca.org.uk

www.empnto.co.uk

www.lantra.co.uk

Index

Notes: Entries refer to the assessment process related to the National Vocational Qualification (NVQ).